AND CHILDBIRTH

For Books for Midwives:

Senior Commissioning Editor: Mary Seager
Development Editor: Catharine Steers
Project Manager: Morven Dean
Design: George Ajayi
Illustration Manager: Bruce Hogarth

HIV

IN PREGNANCY AND CHILDBIRTH

JANE KENNEDY MSc BSc RGN RM

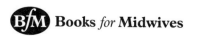
BfM Books *for* Midwives

Books for Midwives
An imprint of Elsevier Science Limited

First edition 1994
Second edition 2003

ISBN 07506 53256

British Library Cataloguing in Publication Data
A catalogue record for this book is available from the British Library

Library of Congress Cataloguing in Publication Data
A catalog record for this book is available from the Library of Congress

Medical knowledge is constantly changing. Standard safety precautions
must be followed, but as new research and clinical experience broaden
our knowledge, changes in treatment and drug therapy may become
necessary or appropriate. Readers are advised to check the most current
product information provided by the manufacturer of each drug to be
administered to verify the recommended dose, the method and duration
of administration, and contraindications. It is the responsibility of the
practitioner, relying on experience and knowledge of the patient, to
determine dosages and the best treatment for each individual patient.
Neither the Publisher nor the author assumes any liability for any injury
and/or damage to persons or property arising from this publication.

ELSEVIER SCIENCE

your source for books,
journals and multimedia
in the health sciences

www.elsevierhealth.com

The
publisher's
policy is to use
**paper manufactured
from sustainable forests**

Printed in China

CONTENTS

Acknowledgements

I could not have written this book without the help and support of many people. I would particularly like to thank:

- All my colleagues in the maternity department (particularly those in the 'laughing office') and multidisciplinary HIV team at Guys and St Thomas' Trust for help and advice and especially Siobhan O'Shea and Ian Chrystie from the Virology section of the Department of Infection.
- My family and friends, who gave me vital encouragement, were a sounding board for ideas and provided food breaks. In particular, my mother, my sister Tessa and friends Sheila, Sarah, Venetia and Dawn.
- Colleagues at Elsevier, particularly Mary and Catharine, who were tolerant of a few deferred deadlines and my ignorance of the world of publishing.
- The HIV positive women who I have worked with over the years and who taught me so much.
- I must acknowledge and thank Caroline Shepherd who wrote the first edition of this book in 1994. She created a resource that has been widely used and referred to by midwives and others involved in pregnancy care, and I am deeply grateful to her for permission to use her initial framework in the preparation for this edition.

Abbreviations used in this text

AIDS   Acquired immune deficiency syndrome

BHIVA   British HIV Association

CD4   Cluster of differentiation antigens type 4 – a molecule on the surface of some lymphocytes onto which HIV can bind

DNA   Deoxyribonucleic acid

EIA   Enzyme immuno-assay

GUM   Genitourinary medicine

HAART   Highly active antiretroviral therapy

HIV   Human immunodeficiency virus

NRTIs   Nucleoside analogue reverse transcriptase inhibitors

NNRTIs   Non-nucleoside reverse transcriptase inhibitors

NtRTIs   Nucleotide analogue reverse transcriptase inhibitors

PCP   Pneumocystis carinii pneumonia

PEP   Post-exposure prophylaxis

PIs   Protease inhibitors

RNA   Ribonucleic acid

UICP   Universal infection control precautions

UKCC   United Kingdom Central Council for Nursing and Midwifery (replaced by Nursing and Midwifery Council from 1st April 2002)

UNAIDS   United Nations AIDS programme

WHO   World Health Organization

Preface to the second edition

Two decades have passed since the first cases of AIDS were described in the medical literature and knowledge has increased significantly since the early descriptions of the retroviruses HIV 1 and HIV 2.*

In particular, advances in knowledge from the mid-1990s have significantly altered the way the condition can be approached and treated.

It is essential for all those involved in maternity care, particularly midwives, obstetricians, general practitioners and other members of the primary health care team, to be aware of the issues women face when considering HIV and pregnancy.

The field of HIV medicine is constantly changing, particularly in the area of antiretroviral therapy and vaccine development, and some of the information in this book will be out of date even before it is printed. Up to date information can be quickly accessed via the Internet and this is an essential source of information for clinical practice in addition to the medical literature and specialist advice.

Whatever changes may take place in the clinical treatment of the HIV positive woman during pregnancy and childbirth, and the subsequent care that she and her baby receive, their physical, social and physiological well-being will always remain the central concern of the professional team that surrounds them.

I hope this book may make a contribution to that concern.

Jane Kennedy 2003

Footnote
*Where the letters HIV are used in the text, this will indicate HIV 1 infection unless otherwise indicated.

Chapter 1

The virus

This chapter will describe the human immunodeficiency virus and provide an overview of the immune system and the effects of the virus upon it. It will also describe the routes of transmission of the virus.

Acquired Immune Deficiency Syndrome (AIDS) was first recognised in 1981.

In 1983, a causative organism, lymphadenopathy virus (LAV), was discovered by Barre-Sinoussi and colleagues (1983), whilst in 1984 human T cell lymphotrophic virus type 3 (HTLV III) was described by a team led by Gallo. Human immunodeficiency virus (HIV 1) became the agreed term later in 1984 for this retrovirus.

HIV is divided into three groups: M, N and O. Group O, identified in the Cameroon in 1994, is extremely rare. In group M there are at least nine sub-types of HIV 1, alphabetically designated, that have so far been described.

The sub-types predominate in different parts of the world, and the occurrence of the same sub-type in countries which are far apart from each other reflects the global dissemination of HIV.

In 1985, another human retrovirus, a variant of HIV 1, was recognised and subsequently named HIV 2. It is less common than HIV 1, and mainly found in patients with West African connections. It appears to be less virulent than HIV 1.

An antibody assay which tests for antibodies to HIV 1 and HIV 2 was developed in 1985 (Adler 2001).

Structure of the virus

Viruses are composed of a core of nucleic acid, made up of the viral genome that consists of either DNA (deoxyribonucleic acid) or RNA (ribonucleic acid), and a protective outer shell made of protein or lipoprotein (the capsid).

HIV is a retrovirus. The genetic building blocks of retroviruses consist of RNA (ribonucleic acid) as opposed to DNA (deoxyribonucleic acid), which is the case in most other organisms. DNA viruses infect host cells and then integrate their DNA into the DNA of the host (this DNA is contained in the nucleus of the cell). As the cell divides, new copies of the viral DNA are made at the same time. These then leave the host cell. RNA viruses must carry out an additional step. They must first make DNA using an enzyme called reverse transcriptase, which is contained in the virus. The resultant DNA is then inserted into the host cell for copying. Once new strands of viral DNA have been copied, the host cell converts the message contained on the DNA into new strands of viral RNA which is packaged in a new viral envelope as the virus leaves the cell.

Retroviruses are so named because their genome encodes the enzyme, reverse transcriptase, which allows DNA to be transcribed from RNA. The most common viral infections found in humans are caused by DNA viruses. Thus HIV can make copies of its own genome as DNA, in host cells such as the human T (thymus derived) lymphocyte carrying the molecule CD4 ('helper').

The proteins in the capsid have an affinity for receptor sites on host cells.

This allows the virus to enter the cell in order to reproduce, as a virus is unable to reproduce outside a host cell (Figure 1.1).

HIV has an outer layer, called the envelope, which develops from the host cell membrane as it buds out from the host cell. Protein molecules called gp (glycoprotein) 41 and gp120 protrude from this envelope and these protein molecules are able to bind to receptors on the CD4 molecule, which is part of the immune system.

The virus life cycle (see Figure 1.1)

The major receptor for HIV is the CD4 surface molecule on T lymphocytes and the envelope protein gp120 virus binds with this. Co-receptors in the immune system are also necessary for virus entry. Receptors and co-receptors enable fusion. The latter function mainly as receptors for chemokines that coordinate the movement, differentiation and function of leucocytes during immune responses. Two receptors, CCR5 and CXCR4, are particularly important. Evidence suggests that CCR5 strains are important for transmission of HIV whilst CXCR4 variants (sometimes known as X4) arise during

Figure 1.1 HIV replication

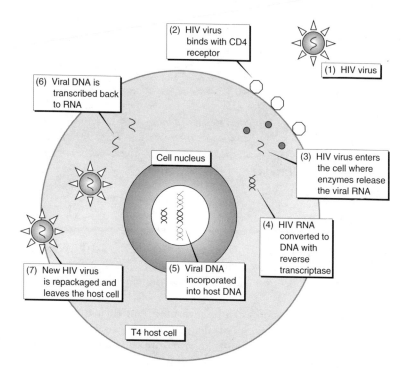

the course of infection (Beverley and Helbert 2001).

CCR5 is widely expressed on lymphocytes, macrophages, dendritic cells and cells of the rectal, vaginal and cervical mucosae.

The reverse transcriptase enables the viral genome to copy itself from RNA to DNA and enter the nucleus of the host cell, becoming incorporated into the DNA of the host cell.

Once incorporated into the host cell, the virus can replicate itself whenever the cell is stimulated to reproduce. The cell now acts as a factory for new viruses.

As the virus production within the cell increases, the cell membrane ruptures, releasing progeny viruses – a process known as budding. The viruses surround themselves with their lipoprotein coat, collected from the cytoplasm of the host cell membrane. These progeny viruses can go on to infect further cells.

CD4 receptors on the T4 lymphocytes and the viral antigens have a high affinity for each other. This leads to many uninfected cells binding to the infected cell and merging with it, forming large bodies called syncitia. A syncitium cannot function, and subsequently dies. Thus although only one T4 cell may have been infected, hundreds of non-infected cells may die with it.

Mortimer and Loveday (2001) have summarised retroviruses thus:

Retroviruses are where the genome of the virus encodes an enzyme, reverse transcriptase, which allows DNA to be transcribed from RNA. Thus HIV can make copies of its own genome, as DNA, in host cells such as the human CD4 lymphocyte (helper). The viral DNA becomes integrated in the lymphocyte genome and this is the basis for chronic HIV infection. (Mortimer and Loveday 2001)

Host responses

As a response to infection, HIV antibodies appear 3-10 weeks after exposure to HIV, and are detectable thereafter, even if the virus has had a damaging effect on lymphocyte function and therefore antibody production.

Neutralising antibodies can be measured, but their titres are low. An inability to mount a neutralising response to HIV antigens, together with the mutability of the virus, are the most likely reasons why conventional approaches to preparing a vaccine have so far failed.

The effects of HIV on the body

To understand how HIV infection causes disease it is essential to have a basic understanding of the immune system and the effect HIV has on immune functioning.

An overview of the immune system

The immune system is comprised of specific and non-specific mechanisms to protect from infectious diseases.

Non-specific immunity consists of the following processes:

● *Prevention* of infection, primarily by intact skin. Each orifice or break in this protection is itself protected by a range of measures such as ciliated cells and mucous membranes, pH changes and chemical secretions, for instance lysozymes in tears.

- *Containment* of infection, either by the process of inflammation or by phagocytosis. In the former, the blood supply containing protective cells and phagocytes is increased to the area exposed to infection. In the latter, bacteria are engulfed and destroyed by white cells including macrophages. In the regions of the body where infectious agents can enter, such as the mouth, anus, genitalia and gut, there are large concentrations of white blood cells in lymph glands.

These mechanisms will often lead to a successful conclusion of infections.

Specific immunity is acquired to afford protection from organisms that may be more hostile or overwhelming. Such immunity may be divided into two types:

- *Humoral immunity* concerns B lymphocytes, which originate from stem cells in the bone marrow. B lymphocytes act on specific antigens. In response to infection, B cells proliferate, become plasma cells, secrete antibody to combine with the antigen and neutralise it, and eventually destroy it. Memory cells are also formed to enable a rapid response to future infection by the same antigen. With HIV, the virus mutates its antigens and therefore memory cells cannot recognise new strains.
- *Cell mediated immunity* concerns T (thymus derived) lymphocytes that also originate from stem cells. They have differing but interlinked functions provided by helper cells and suppressor cells and require a specific growth factor called interleukin 2. When T lymphocytes carrying the surface molecule CD4, known as CD4 lymphocytes or T helper cells, are stimulated by contact with an antigen they respond by cell division and the production of lymphokines, such as interferons, interleukins, tumour necrosis factor and chemokines. Lymphokines act as local hormones controlling the growth, maturation and behaviour of other lymphocytes particularly the cytotoxic/suppressor (CD8) T cells and antibody producing B lymphocytes. Lymphokines also affect the maturation and function of monocytes, tissue macrophages and dendritic cells. Macrophages and particularly dendritic cells are important antigen-presenting cells for initiating the immune responses of lymphocytes. Not only do they act as a reservoir for the virus but also their antigen presenting function is impaired, with secondary effects on lymphocytes.

CD4 (helper) is present on a large proportion of monocytes and macrophages, Langerhan's cells of the skin, and dendritic cells of all tissues.

CD8 (suppressor) cells are produced to stop the immune reaction going out of control. They inhibit the helper, cytotoxic and lymphokine-producing cells. The normal ratio of CD4:CD8 cells is 2:1 and if this ratio is disturbed this will lead to a lowered response to infection.

Figure 1.2   Specific immunity

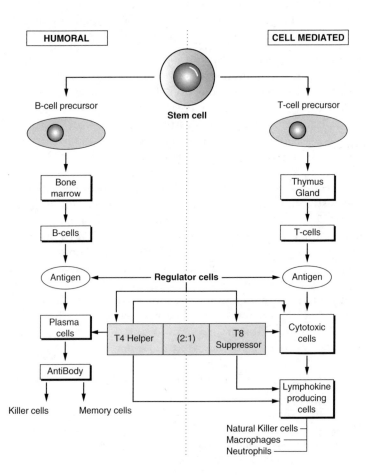

The effects of HIV on the immune system

With regard to HIV infection, it is the role of the T lymphocytes that is vital to understanding the mechanism by which HIV causes disease, particularly the role of T (helper) CD4 lymphocytes which interact with CD8 T (killer) lymphocytes and B lymphocytes in the response to antigens.

Some have found it useful to visualise CD4 lymphocytes as the 'leader of the immunological orchestra', with their pivotal role in the immune response and their destruction helping to explain the immunosuppressive effect of the virus (Beverley and Helbert 2001).

Once HIV has entered the CD4 cell, it remains there until the cell is stimulated to reproduce, and once activated, will produce virus and will itself be destroyed. Due to their reduced numbers the CD4 helper cells are less able to perform their normal function as part of the human immune response.

There are two types of immune response: primary and secondary. A primary response takes place when the immune system encounters an antigen for the first time; a secondary one when an individual has previously raised a response to a particular foreign organism. Both these responses are damaged by infection with HIV which may lead to opportunistic infections that reactivate, or to tumours in advanced HIV disease and immune suppression (e.g. Kaposi's sarcoma).

Though individuals may remain healthy for long periods, a feature of disease progression, often prior to the development of new clinical symptoms, is a fall in the number of CD4 lymphocytes, and in advanced disease, the number of CD8 cells also falls.

Therefore, as an epidemiological review published by the Communicable Disease Surveillance Centre (CDSC) explains:

... in the natural course of the infection and disease, without antiretroviral drug therapy or other interventions, the virus causes progressive immuno-suppression by selectively destroying the CD4 lymphocyte set and thereby predisposes infected individuals to a characteristic group of opportunistic infections and malignancies. (CDSC 2001)

Transmission of the virus

The virus is primarily blood borne although it has been isolated in other body fluids including semen, vaginal and cervical secretions, tears, saliva, cerebrospinal fluid and breast milk.

The main routes of transmission are:

- Sexual (often described as horizontal transmission).
- Mother to baby transmission (also known as vertical transmission).
- Contaminated intravenous drug using equipment.
- Blood borne transmission via infected blood, blood products, infected human organs (if used in transplantation) or infected donor semen (if used in artificial insemination procedures). Such transmission would also include cases of occupational infection and/or other transmission via contaminated medical equipment.

Sexual (horizontal) transmission

Globally, unprotected sexual intercourse, whether heterosexual or homosexual, is the main route of transmission. It is estimated that more than 80% of HIV infections are transmitted by heterosexual intercourse.

However, HIV is not automatically transmitted every time sexual intercourse takes place, and the infectivity rate per occurrence of sexual contact is approximately 0.3% (i.e. 3 per 1000).

For transmission to occur requires sexual contact involving the exchange of body fluids or blood-to-blood contact. Virus is shed from infected individuals into both the ejaculate and cervico-vaginal fluids. In spermatozoa, the adherence of HIV to it and the incorporation of HIV DNA within it, are believed to be factors in transmission. Both cell-free and cell-associated virus in the reproductive fluids appear to be infectious, and heterosexual transmission most probably occurs through direct contact with such virus present in the genital tract (Royce 1997).

In women, the flora and fauna of the vagina are affected by a number of factors including age, contraceptive practices, sexual excitement and intercourse, bleeding including menses, differences in host susceptibility and other systemic diseases, and these may affect transmission of HIV (Alexander 1996).

The presence of other sexually transmitted infections can also act as a co-factor for transmission of HIV, and this may be due to the presence of genital ulcers, induced immuno-supression, or receptors on the pathogens. These infections include genital ulcers (chancroid, herpes simplex and syphilis), gonorrhoea and chlamydia, and possibly bacterial vaginosis, human papilloma virus infection and candidiasis. It is therefore important that such infections are treated promptly when they occur in men and women to reduce the chance of HIV transmission.

Such infections may also make an individual susceptible to sexual transmission of HIV, hence the need for prompt treatment of both partners.

A randomised controlled trial demonstrated that treatment of sexually transmitted infections reduced HIV incidence by approximately 40% (Grosskurth et al 1995).

Other factors which can influence an individual's susceptibility to sexually acquired infection include the type of unprotected sexual intercourse, with receptive penile-anal intercourse representing a significant risk for men and women. Since the rectal mucosa is thin, lesions may occur during intercourse, increasing the chances of transmission. Anal sex has mainly been considered as the route of transmission in homosexual men but studies have indicated that at least 25% of women in the United States may, even if only occasionally, engage in anal intercourse (Reinisch 1995).

The risk of transmission from oral sex has been difficult to quantify as many couples engage in other sexual activities as well. Other factors such as bleeding gums or a high viral load may be significant. Although such transmission cannot be ruled out, its likelihood is considered to be very rare (Alexander 1996, Romero 2002).

Other factors which appear to affect the risk of acquiring HIV through sexual transmission are age (with the risk being greater for individuals aged over 45 years, and for women who are young when they become sexually active), and whether or not a man is circumcised (Royce 1997).

Additionally, if the individual has recently acquired HIV or has advanced disease, which may be indicated by a high viral load, this is likely to affect transmission. Virus shedding in the genital tract occurs during times of viraemia, such as in the initial infection stages, and appears to be related to plasma HIV 1 RNA levels (Kovacs et al 2001). Therefore antiviral therapy may decrease infectivity by reducing viral shedding.

Early studies suggested that male to female transmission was more efficient than female to male transmission, quoting rates of 15% and 8% respectively. However, more recent evidence suggests that transmission may occur with equal frequency and depends on the factors described earlier in this chapter (Quinn et al 2000).

Additionally, though the number of documented woman to woman transmissions is small, female partners of HIV infected women should receive appropriate prevention advice regarding avoidance of potentially infectious secretions (White 1997).

Strategies for the prevention of sexual HIV transmission need to take account of all these factors if they are to achieve any success. The condom can provide protection against infection and pregnancy. Condoms lubricated with spermicides containing Nonoxynol-9, which has been shown to inactivate HIV, can provide extra protection if the condom breaks. However, Nonoxynol-9 has also been reported to cause irritation of the genital tract lining, which can increase the risk of entry of any virus present.

Recommending the regular and correct use of condoms during sexual intercourse, and the prompt, appropriate treatment of sexually transmitted infections is vital.

Additionally, health promotion campaigns that encourage individuals not to be pressurised into early or unwanted sexual intercourse, or endorse the idea that men and women should reduce their number of sexual partners, are important.

However, all of these strategies need to be seen within their social and cultural context. Peer pressure, cultural expectations or financial considerations may mean that an individual takes part in sexual behaviour that puts him or her at risk of HIV infection. Thus health promotion strategies need to be broad and to look at a number of issues such as empowerment, peer support, cultural and financial considerations.

For example, there is evidence that consistent and correct use of condoms is highly effective in preventing the transmission of HIV. The European Study Group on Heterosexual Transmission of HIV conducted a study of discordant couples, where one was HIV positive and the other HIV negative, looking at condom use and transmission of HIV. Of the 124 couples that used condoms consistently, none of the HIV sero-negative partners became infected with HIV despite a total of about 15,000 episodes of intercourse (European Study Group on Heterosexual Transmission of HIV 1994).

However, if condoms are unaffordable, unavailable or unacceptable then they will not be used to prevent transmission of HIV.

Mother to baby (vertical) transmission

Mother to infant transmission can occur either transplacentally, perinatally or during breast feeding. This route of transmission will be explored later (see Chapter 4).

Intravenous drug use

Eight per cent of HIV infections in the United Kingdom, diagnosed by the end of 2000, had been attributed to injecting drug use (Department of Health 2001a).

In the early 1980s in parts of Scotland, such as Edinburgh and Dundee, there was rapid HIV spread through injecting drug use and the shared use of equipment.

Harm reduction initiatives, such as needle exchange programmes and methadone maintenance regimes were initiated by the mid-1980s in other parts of the United Kingdom to try to prevent the transmission of infection via this route. In addition, services developed which acknowledged the links between intravenous drug use and commercial sex work; that is, men and women undertaking the latter in order to fund their drug-using habit. Such services included improving the availability of condoms in conjunction with needle exchanges and other infection prevention advice. Such strategies appear to have had some level of success and this may be one of the reasons that HIV transmission from injecting drug use has had a smaller contribution to the epidemic in parts of the United Kingdom than in other developed countries such as Italy, Portugal and Spain.

However, it is important not to be complacent about injecting drug use as a route for transmission of any blood borne virus, including HIV. There has been evidence of rapid spread of HIV related to intravenous drug use in several countries of the former Soviet Union, and in Thailand, and large outbreaks have been reported amongst intravenous drug users in Canada (CDSC 2001, UNAIDS 2001).

In the United Kingdom, rates of shared needle/syringe use increased in the late 1990s, with one third of intravenous drug users reporting direct sharing of needles and syringes (Department of Health 2000a).

Blood borne transmission

Transmission via blood transfusion or infected blood products is less common now, since many countries have implemented universal screening of donors and heat-treatment of blood products. In the United Kingdom, men and women who believe they may be at risk of having a blood borne infection, including HIV, are asked not to donate blood. Universal screening of all blood donors and heat treatment of blood products was introduced in 1985.

Since that time, there have been no recorded cases of transmission via clotting factor concentrates and there have been only two proven incidents of blood infectious for HIV being accepted for transfusion in the United Kingdom.

The contaminated blood was donated in the donor's 'window period' of infection (CDSC 2001). Thus when individuals require blood or blood products for clinical care they should be reassured appropriately about the safety of such products.

However, if countries do not have the economic or laboratory resources to screen all blood donors, or if commercial blood donation is practised without stringent screening measures, contaminated blood as a route of infection will remain a problem. This has been demonstrated in parts of sub-Saharan Africa and south Asia (Grant and De Cock 2001).

Infection screening, including for HIV, is required for all organ and tissue donors. The Human Fertilisation and Embryology Authority (HFEA) requires that all egg or sperm donors should be screened for blood borne viruses, including HIV (HFEA 2001). If infection is detected, the organ or tissue is not used and there are not believed to have been any cases of transmission via this route in the United Kingdom since such screening was implemented.

Although rare, there have been instances of transmission via the use of non-sterile medical equipment. In a case that received attention in the early 1990s, several hundred children in Romania were found to be infected with HIV following the use of contaminated needles in vaccination programmes or from the use of infected, pooled plasma.

Occupational transmission, that is transmission to health care workers through injury at work, is also rare but can occur. Issues for practice are examined in Chapter 9.

Prevention of HIV transmission

Effective strategies to reduce the spread of HIV need to address all the routes of transmission. These include:

- Using condoms for all penetrative sexual intercourse
- Reducing number of sexual partners and delaying the age at which first sexual intercourse takes place
- Effective screening for and prompt treatment of sexually transmitted infections
- Adopting appropriate interventions to reduce mother to infant transmission

- Supporting safer drug-using practices including not sharing equipment used for injection drug use
- Screening of all blood and organ donors and appropriate treatment of all blood products.

Work is currently in progress regarding the development of a preventive vaccine either to protect against HIV or to modify the course of the disease. The traditional approaches in vaccine development of using a weakened strain of the virus (also known as live attenuated vaccine), or an extract of cell cultured virus (killed virus) are generally considered too dangerous for HIV. However, a recombinant vaccine based on the protein gp120 is being used in clinical trials as well as more complex vaccine systems. Although some of the work appears promising, there is still much more research to be done in this area (WHO-UNAIDS HIV Vaccine Initiative) and vaccine development will not be a replacement for other prevention strategies previously described.

Summary

Human immunodeficiency virus (HIV) is a human retrovirus, prevalent globally and transmitted in four principal ways:

- Sexually
- From mother to baby
- By injecting drug use
- From infected blood and blood products.

The virus causes progressive immuno-suppression and this leads to infected individuals being susceptible to a group of opportunistic infections and malignancies. Despite significant advances in treatment, the infection remains incurable and predominantly affects younger adults, with serious consequences for all aspects of society.

Heterosexual intercourse is the commonest route of transmission.

Though HIV prevalence varies around the world, all countries have been affected by this infection. Whilst the development of an effective vaccine is awaited, other strategies regarding prevention of transmission need to be adopted. These include:

- Using condoms for all penetrative sexual intercourse
- Reducing number of sexual partners and delaying the age at which

first sexual intercourse takes place
- Effective screening for and prompt treatment of sexually transmitted infections
- Adopting appropriate interventions to reduce mother to infant transmission
- Safer drug using practices including not sharing equipment used for injection drug use
- Screening of all blood and organ donors and appropriate treatment of all blood products.

Chapter 2

Global epidemiology

HIV has had a worldwide impact and there are virtually no areas that have not reported cases of infection. As of December 2001, an estimated 40 million people are living with HIV/AIDS. These include 2.7 million children less than fifteen years of age and 17.6 million women.

A total of 5 million people are believed to have been newly infected with HIV during 2001, including 1.8 million women and 800,000 children under 15 years of age. The total number of AIDS deaths in 2001 was 3 million, including 1.1 million women and around 580,000 children. Since the beginning of the epidemic, more than 20 million people have died of AIDS.

The worst affected continent is Africa, but other regions are seeing increasing levels of infection, such as parts of Asia and the Caribbean. Whilst significant levels of transmission are from unprotected heterosexual intercourse, injecting drug use remains an important route for infection to spread in areas such as Eastern Europe and Central Asia (UNAIDS 2001).

Table 2.1 shows the breakdown of estimated numbers per region. It is important to relate these figures to total population numbers: in sub-Saharan Africa more than 8% of the population are infected, whilst in North America, Western Europe and Australia and New Zealand it is less than 1% of the population.

A number of factors are believed to have influenced the patterns of the HIV epidemic globally. Within sub-Saharan Africa, the relationship between sexually transmitted infections, parasitic diseases, tuberculosis and HIV, against a background of widespread poverty and inadequate health care, has influenced the nature of the epidemic in many African countries. It is important to be aware that the situation may differ

Table 2.1 Estimated number of people living with HIV/AIDS, end 2001

Region	Number of people infected	Estimated prevalence (%)
Sub-Saharan Africa	28,100,000	8.57
East Asia & Pacific	1,000,000	0.06
Australia & New Zealand	15,200	0.13
South & South East Asia	6,100,000	0.54
Eastern Europe & Central Asia	1,000,000	0.21
Western Europe	560,000	0.23
North Africa & Middle East	440,000	0.12
North America	940,000	0.58
Caribbean	420,000	2.11
Latin America	1,400,000	0.49
Global total	**39,975,200**	**1.07**

Source: www.unaids.org/epidemic_update/report/table

Table 2.2

Country	Numbers living with HIV/AIDS	Estimated adult prevalence (%)
Botswana	290,000	36.0
Zimbabwe	1,500,000	25.0
Swaziland	130,000	25.0
Lesotho	240,000	24.0
Namibia	160,000	20.0
Zambia	870,000	20.0
South Africa	4,200,000	19.9
Kenya	2,100,000	14.0
Ethiopia	3,000,000	10.0
Tanzania	1,300,000	8.0
Nigeria	2,700,000	5.0

Source: www.unaids.org/epidemic_update/report/table

from one country to another, as Africa is a continent of more than 50 countries. According to UNAIDS estimates, HIV has hit certain countries the hardest (see Table 2.2). However, there are examples of reductions in prevalence rates, such as in Uganda, where, following early and extensive prevention work, the rate has fallen from about 14% in the early 1990s to about 8%. There are also indications in Zambia to suggest that rates of HIV among pregnant 15 to 19-year-olds in the capital, Lusaka, have fallen from 28% to about 14%.

Clearly such strategies need to be sustained and resourced in order to reduce the impact of this epidemic on every aspect of African society. The impact is reflected in the figures for AIDS orphans, children who have lost their mother or both their parents. Such children are usually raised by grandparents or siblings and the latter are usually children themselves. Current estimates for the cumulative number of AIDS orphans since the epidemic began are more than 12 million for sub-Saharan Africa. The epidemic has had an effect on many aspects of life including economically, with a reduction in the numbers of workers available (through illness and death) and diversion of resources to health care needs, and educationally, where children leave school earlier as their parents die.

It has been estimated that HIV in Africa claims more lives than war. During 1998, 200,000 people died as a result of war in sub-Saharan Africa; 2,000,000 died from AIDS (UNAIDS 2001).

In comparison to sub-Saharan Africa, the HIV prevalence in other regions of the world is lower (see Table 2.1), though as such figures are generally estimates, there are concerns about the adequacy of the surveillance systems in some areas.

However, HIV is having an impact in all regions of the world.

In South and South East Asia, whilst prevalence rates may only exceed 1% in three countries (Thailand, Cambodia and Myanmar) this may be misleading as a number of Asian countries have large populations. This can mean that there may be more people living with HIV in such countries than in many African countries. For example, only 7 people in 1,000 are HIV positive in India but because of the size of the population, this equates to an estimated 3.86 million people – the second largest HIV positive population in one country in the world (UNAIDS 2001).

In parts of north-east India, widespread injecting drug use helped to spread HIV infection, whilst a different pattern was seen in southern and western states with prevalence levels of 25-71% amongst sex workers in cities including New Delhi, Hyderabad, Vellore and Mumbai. In Thailand, 2.15% of the population were believed to be HIV positive at the end of 2001, and the main route of transmission is heterosexual sex, although there is evidence of continuing transmission related to injecting drug use. Cambodia has a significant HIV epidemic, though, like Thailand, it has undertaken a very active programme of HIV prevention despite a lack of resources. Campaigns encouraging condom use, particularly among men using sex workers, have seen their reported use increase dramatically between 1997 and 1999. There have also been signs of a decline in HIV rates among pregnant women, from 3.2% in 1997 to 2.3% in 2000 (UNAIDS 2001).

The worst affected countries in East Asia and the Pacific are believed to be China, Japan and Papua New Guinea. With China's vast population, there is evidence of a rising heterosexual epidemic, highlighted by a significant recent increase in sexually transmitted infections. There has also been a noted spread of HIV among blood and plasma donors, particularly in central China, as a result of alleged medical malpractice. As well as the impact on the infected individuals, there are concerns that the effect of this issue may also hinder health promotion and HIV prevention campaigns because of communities' distrust of 'the authorities' and their health messages (UNAIDS 2001).

The epidemics in Eastern Europe and Central Asia are considered to be some of the fastest growing in the world, strongly affected by rising rates of injecting drug use. Particularly affected are the Ukraine, Belarus, the Republic of Moldova and the Russian Federation. In the latter, new infections have increased by 305% from 1999 to the first half of 2000 (UNAIDS 2001).

The HIV epidemic continues to grow in Latin America, with significantly affected countries including Mexico, Argentina, Guyana, Belize and Brazil.

In Central America, HIV is predominantly spread by heterosexual transmission; in Brazil there are also high rates among men who have sex with men and injecting drug users. However, the Brazilian government has undertaken HIV prevention campaigns that have shown some success, particularly with drug users, and it is committed to providing free antiretroviral treatment to all those who need it. AIDS deaths have almost halved since the introduction of this policy in 1996. Reported condom use amongst men who have sex with men increased significantly during the early 1990s. Nevertheless, in poorer parts of Brazil, few prevention activities are reportedly taking place, and levels of unprotected sex remain high.

The proportion of the population who are HIV infected in the Caribbean, approximately 2% of all adults, is higher than in any other region outside Africa. The focus of the epidemic is among heterosexuals, and sex between men and women is the main route of transmission. There are believed to be two significant factors behind this heterosexual epidemic: the early initiation of sexual relationships, and the high turnover of sexual partners common among young people (UNAIDS 2001). The worst affected countries in this region are Haiti, the Dominican Republic, the Bahamas, and Trinidad &

Tobago where between 1.05% and 5.17% of the adult population are living with HIV/AIDS.

Within North America the availability of antiretroviral treatment has led to a decline in death rates. The transmission of HIV is concentrated more and more among ethnic minority populations. For example, African-Americans make up 12% of the population of the United States, but represented 47% of reported AIDS cases in 2000. There is evidence from surveys in the United States that risk behaviour is increasing amongst some groups and in certain ages (UNAIDS 2001).

Within Western Europe there has also been a reduction of AIDS incidence following the introduction of antiretroviral therapy. The epidemic has been mainly concentrated among men who have sex with men, but several countries have reported an increase in the number of heterosexual transmissions since the mid-1990s. Many of the heterosexually acquired HIV cases occurred in persons with links to countries where the HIV epidemic has become more established amongst the general population.

Some Western European countries continue to have high prevalence rates among injecting drug users. A recent study in Barcelona showed that 51% of injecting drug users were HIV positive. The worst affected countries are France, Spain, Italy and Portugal (UNAIDS 2001).

In Australia and New Zealand the epidemic appears to be largely confined to men who have sex with men. As has been demonstrated in other countries there is evidence emerging that, following the introduction of antiretroviral treatments, people are becoming less concerned about HIV infection and thus more prepared to engage in unprotected sexual intercourse (UNAIDS 2001).

In summary, the picture of the epidemic around the world has some similar features. These include associations between poverty and risk behaviour for HIV, injecting drug use and a rise in sexually transmitted infections in parallel with a rise in HIV infections. However, lessons can be learnt from areas where strategies such as increased condom use and safer drug-using initiatives have been implemented and have shown some success in reducing HIV transmission.

The picture in the United Kingdom

Since the infection was first noted in the early 1980s its prevalence and transmission have been monitored by a number of agencies working in collaboration. The Public Health Laboratory Service (PHLS) Communicable Disease Surveillance Centre, the Scottish Centre for Infection and Environmental Health, The Institute for Child Health (London) and the Oxford Haemophilia Centre, as well as individual clinics and centres, have all contributed to the Unlinked Anonymised Surveillance programme for HIV/AIDS and other infections in the United Kingdom.

As a result of such collaboration, there is a relatively clear picture of the pattern of the epidemic in the United Kingdom. Various groups who are at risk of HIV infection are included in the surveys: men who have sex with men, heterosexuals, injecting drug users, blood and blood factor recipients, children born to HIV infected mothers, commercial sex workers, prisoners and health care workers. Reports are regularly produced about various aspects of the infection that may influence policy and practice. There has been a review of the epidemic in the United Kingdom from its beginnings to 2000 (CDSC 2001).

From 1982 to the end of 2001, 48,226 people have been diagnosed with HIV infection and their infection confidentially notified.

Table 2.3 HIV infected individuals* by year of first reported UK** diagnosis: UK data to end December 2001

How infection was probably acquired	<1992	1992	1993	1994	1995	1996	1997	1998	1999	2000	2001	Total
Sex between men***	12774	1639	1498	1479	1466	1538	1389	1341	1321	1429	1095	26969
Sex between men and women	2253	780	766	793	848	837	1003	1150	1396	1867	1758	13451
Injecting drug use	2300	187	202	168	182	172	168	129	109	101	71	3789
Blood products e.g. for haemophilia	1353	9	4	3	4	3	2	2	3	3	2	1388
Blood/tissue transfer	143	14	13	14	16	18	26	8	16	19	14	301
Mother to infant	116	57	67	63	59	60	83	92	75	91	18	781
Other/undetermined	528	53	63	47	61	55	50	68	94	144	384	1547
Total	19467	2739	2613	2567	2636	2683	2721	2790	3014	3654	3342	48226

* individuals with laboratory reports of infection, or with AIDS or death reported but no matching laboratory report numbers, particularly for recent years, will rise as further reports are received
** includes 68 individuals first reported from the Channel Islands or the Isle of Man
*** includes 664 men who also injected drugs
Source: Communicable Disease Report Weekly (CDR) 31/01/02 (PHLS)

Table 2.4 Estimated prevalent HIV infections, diagnosed and undiagnosed, among adults* in the UK at the end of 2000 (rounded to nearest 100)

Route of infection	Number diagnosed**	Number undiagnosed (% of total)***	Total
Sex between men	13800	3200 (19%)	17000
Injecting drug use males and females	1300	200 (13%)	1500
Sex between men and women – male	3300	3100 (48%)	6400
Sex between men and women – female	5200	2900 (36%)	8100
Sex between men and women – total	8500	6000 (41%)	14500
Blood products**** males and females	500	0 (0%)	500
Grand total	**24100**	**9400 (28%)**	**33500**

* includes adults aged 16 years and over and excludes those who have died during the year
** diagnosed numbers were obtained from SOPHID (Survey of prevalent diagnosed HIV infections) and SCIEH (Scottish Centre for Infection and Environmental Health) and were adjusted for under-reporting and failure to access services
*** undiagnosed numbers were derived using data from SOPHID, NATSSAL 2000 (National Survey of Sexual Attitudes and Lifestyles), and the UAPMP (Unlinked Anonymous Prevalence Monitoring Programme). undiagnosed numbers for the United Kingdom were derived by scaling up the England and Wales data
**** all cases infected by blood and blood products or tissue were assumed to be diagnosed
Source: CDR weekly 31/01/02

18,334 had a report of AIDS; 12,287 (67%) of them had died, and 2,263 with no report of AIDS had also died (5%).

Table 2.3 illustrates the pattern of routes of infection in the United Kingdom.

At the end of 2000, an estimated 33,500 adults aged 16 years and over were living with HIV in the United Kingdom; 9,400 (28%) of whom were seemingly unaware of their infection.

The highest proportion of undiagnosed infection was in the category of heterosexual infection (Table 2.4).

Among new infections in the previous year, the proportion infected through sex between men and women has increased from 29% (5,506) in 1999 to 31% (6,762) in 2000. A higher proportion of female heterosexuals with HIV were diagnosed than males: 64% compared to 52%. This may be attributed to antenatal screening (PHLS 2002).

Prevalence amongst pregnant women has been monitored by the anonymous unlinked surveys since the late 1980s. Prevalence of HIV infection in London in 2000 was 1:350 overall, the highest level recorded so far and significantly higher in inner rather than in outer London. HIV prevalence varied substantially according to maternal district of residence within London from zero to 1:140.

Elsewhere in England, although the prevalence has remained low, it rose in the late 1990s from 1:6,500 to 1:3,700 in 2000. Likewise, in Scotland HIV prevalence has doubled from 0.023% in 1999 to 0.047% in 2000 (Department of Health 2001a).

During the 1990s there was considerable public health concern about low rates of detection of HIV infection in pregnancy. As women were unaware of their infection, they were unable to access treatments for their own health or take up interventions that had been shown to reduce vertical transmission. National targets for HIV testing and detection of infection were issued in 1999, and are discussed further elsewhere. Following their implementation, the numbers of women being diagnosed before and during pregnancy has increased. During 2000, in inner London, an estimated 82% of maternal HIV infections were diagnosed before delivery: in outer London the equivalent figure was 65% and in the rest of England 56%.

In inner London, the proportion of infections first diagnosed during antenatal care also increased from 54% in 1999 to 70% in 2000. A rise was also seen, over the same time period, in the rest of England from 11% to 41% (Department of Health 2001a).

With more women having a diagnosis made in the antenatal period, the opportunities for accessing interventions to reduce vertical transmission have increased. This in turn has led to a declining number of reported cases of infection in infants.

Summary

- HIV has had a worldwide impact and there are virtually no areas that have not reported cases of infection.
- Since the beginning of the epidemic, more than 20 million people have died of AIDS.

- The worst affected continent is Africa but other regions are seeing increasing levels of infection such as parts of Asia and the Caribbean.
- Whilst significant levels of transmission are from unprotected heterosexual intercourse, injecting drug use remains an important route for infection to spread in areas such as Eastern Europe and Central Asia (UNAIDS 2001).
- HIV/AIDS contributes significantly to rising adult and child mortality rates in many countries.

Chapter 3

The course of HIV disease

This chapter will examine the course of HIV infection in adults and disease progression including the effect of antiretroviral therapy. Significant change has occurred in recent years in the management of this disease and it is important to have an understanding of this process when providing care for infected women and their families.

Classification of disease

The definition of Acquired Immune Deficiency Syndrome (AIDS) has altered over the years in line with increasing awareness of the wide range of clinical manifestations relating to infection with HIV. At present, AIDS is defined as an illness identified with one or more specific diseases (see Appendix 1).

If no other causes of immune deficiency are present, certain diagnosed diseases are also suggestive of AIDS (see Appendix 1).

Four different stages of HIV disease in adults have been described and were classified by the Centres for Disease Control (CDC) in the United States in 1992. This classification system (CDC 1992) is based on a number of factors including the presence of clinical signs and symptoms of disease, the presence of certain conditions and investigative findings and the degree of immuno-suppression as indicated by the CD4 lymphocyte count.

- Group I – Primary HIV infection (seroconversion)
- Group II – Asymptomatic HIV infection
- Group III – Persistent generalised lymphadenopathy
- Group IV – Symptomatic HIV infection

Group IV is commonly sub-divided to reflect the different phases of symptomatic infection including opportunistic infections, cancers and constitutional disease that are AIDS defining.

Group I – Primary HIV infection (seroconversion)

This is the stage following infection with HIV during which antibodies develop. This takes up to three months, though antibodies have most commonly developed by between four to six weeks after infection. During primary HIV infection, there is sometimes a high rate of viral replication, leading to a rise in the HIV viral load and a fall in the CD4 count, though this may only be for a short period.

Individuals may present with symptoms at the time of seroconversion but this is not always the case. Mindel and Tenant-Flowers (2001) state that only 25-65% of people have been found to present with symptoms at the time of primary HIV infection.

Box 3.1   Signs and symptoms of primary HIV infection

- Glandular fever like illness
- Fever, malaise, diarrhoea, neuralgia
- Arthralgia, sore throat, headaches
- Lymphadenopathy
- Macular papular rash
- Ulceration of oropharynx or anogenital area
- Neurological symptoms: meningitis, neuropathy, myelopathy, encephalopathy

---

However the severe symptoms are rare and the mild symptoms may vary so a diagnosis at this stage may be overlooked. Appropriate diagnostic tests, including HIV antibody testing and HIV PCR may be used at this time.

Information on diagnostic testing is explored further in Chapter 5.

Treatment at this stage of the disease is mainly aimed at the symptoms individuals present with. However it has been suggested that using antiretroviral therapy at this time may be more effective because the virus may be relatively susceptible, due to the low levels that would be capable of replication. However this option has to be balanced against future consideration of antiviral therapy and whether early commencement of antiviral therapy could influence the development of resistant virus that could restrict future treatment choices (Mindel and Tenant-Flowers 2001).

Group II – Asymptomatic infection

Even in the absence of antiviral therapy, this stage of infection can persist for ten or more years. HIV antibodies can still be detected in infected individuals but the amount of virus in blood and lymphoid tissues falls and the rate of HIV replication is slower than at other stages of the disease. CD4 lymphocyte counts are generally within normal ranges and above 350 cells/mm^3.

During this phase many individuals are clinically asymptomatic and therefore, if they do not believe they have been at risk of infection, may be less likely to seek diagnostic antibody testing.

Group III – Persistent generalised lymphadenopathy

An HIV positive individual may present with persistent generalised lymphadenopathy but be otherwise well. The lymphadenopathy appears to persist for at least a few months and is not due to any other cause such as other infections, tumours or sarcoidosis which should be excluded when making a diagnosis. The presence of lymphadenopathy due to HIV does not appear to make the prognosis poorer.

Group IV – Symptomatic HIV infection

In clinical settings, the terms symptomatic HIV infection or advanced HIV disease are used more widely than the term AIDS to define an individual's stage of disease.

Group IV is divided into a number of sub-sections:

- IV – Symptomatic HIV infection
- IVA – HIV wasting syndrome (AIDS) and constitutional disease
- IVB – HIV encephalopathy (AIDS) and neurological disease
- IVC1 – Major opportunistic infections specified as AIDS defining
- IVC2 – Minor opportunistic infections
- IVD – Cancers specified as AIDS defining
- IVE – Other conditions.

The infected individual may suffer from a number of symptoms as the HIV infection progresses, including malaise, fevers, night sweats, weight loss, skin and mouth problems and haematological disorders. Many of these can be treated or their symptoms alleviated, and may

Table 3.1 Centres for Disease Control classification system for HIV disease 1993

Classification	CD4 count x 10⁶/l >500 (1)	CD4 count x 10⁶/l 200-499 (2)	CD4 count x 10⁶/l <199 (3)
A Asymptomatic including Groups I, II & III	A1	A2	A3
B Symptomatic not A or C	B1	B2	B3
C AIDS defining conditions	C1	C2	C3

be completely resolved if antiretroviral therapies are commenced.

The different sub-divisions of symptomatic HIV infection include a wide range of conditions that may be present in association with immune deficiency.

These include neurological disease, opportunistic infections such as Pneumocystis carinii pneumonia (PCP), toxoplasmosis and cytomegalovirus, and cancers including non-Hodgkin's lymphoma, cervical carcinoma and Kaposi's sarcoma, though the latter is rare in women (Adler 2001).

In 1993 this classification system was further modified and is widely used at present (Table 3.1).

Additionally, in 1993, the CDC included all HIV infected persons with CD4 lymphocyte counts less than 200 cells/mm³ as fulfilling a definition of an AIDS diagnosis, though the use of this classification has not been widely adopted outside of the United States of America (CDC 1992, PHLS 1993).

The criteria have been revised in the United States (CDC 1999).

In many countries, including the United Kingdom, AIDS remains a clinical diagnosis defined by at least one indicator disease.

There may be overlap in some of these definitions, so classifying an individual's stage of disease cannot always be an exact science.

Many of these definitions require access to complex laboratory investigations and their results, and these are not available in all parts of the world. Therefore, the World Health Organization (WHO) has introduced clinical case definitions for AIDS that can be used in such settings (Grant and De Cock 2001).

The course of disease in HIV infection

In an average patient, without antiretroviral therapy, the time from infection with HIV to AIDS is approximately ten years (Mindel and Tenant-Flowers 2001). As the disease progresses, there is a reduction in immune competence with CD4 cells declining by approximately $50/mm^3$ per year as a result of reduced production. This follows increased replication of HIV from areas where it has been dormant, though what activates the HIV to replicate is uncertain.

An infected individual's prognosis is likely to be poorer if they have a steeper decline in their CD4 count and a higher viral load. The average viral load, without antiretroviral therapy, is 30,000-50,000 copies per millilitre.

Other factors that are believed to influence the speed of disease progression include whether the individual received a large inoculum of virus prior to infection (for example, from a contaminated blood transfusion where the donor had a high viral load). Also, if an individual had a symptomatic primary HIV infection or was of an older age at diagnosis, this has been associated with rapid disease progression (Darby et al 1996).

There appears to be no difference between men and women in relation to disease progression (Newman 1998) though earlier studies had indicated that women had a shorter disease course and a more rapid decline. This was subsequently explained more by psychosocial factors, such as differences between men and women in access to medical care, than by biological ones.

Psychosocial factors, including issues relating to disclosure of status and matters associated with mental, physical and reproductive health, are equally important for women with HIV disease (Sherr 1997).

However, some patients remain asymptomatic without antiretroviral treatment, with CD4 counts in the normal range, at 7-10 years following infection. Such patients are sometimes termed 'long term non-progressors'.

HIV 2 infection

HIV 2 infection appears to have a slower but similar course to HIV 1 infection. There has been evidence of higher levels of CD4 counts in HIV 2 infection than in HIV 1 and a lower incidence of falling CD4 counts (Markovitz 1993, van der Ende et al 1996). Heterosexual spread of HIV 2 appears to be slower than HIV 1 (Kanki et al 1994) and relatively small numbers have been reported within the United Kingdom (Department of Health 2001a). Many aspects of management of HIV 2 infection are similar to those for HIV 1.

Management of HIV I disease

Management of the disease in an individual will initially be dependent on the stage of the infection at which he or she is diagnosed. If diagnosed in the asymptomatic stage, decisions about treatment and care would be very different than for someone diagnosed with advanced, symptomatic HIV disease. Regular clinical monitoring is recommended for all infected individuals, particularly those with a steeply declining CD4 count, a CD4 count less than 350, those with a high viral load, or those who are symptomatic.

In the United Kingdom, following diagnosis the initial assessment for the infected individual should include a full medical history and examination as well as a number of serological tests if possible. Two tests, the CD4 lymphocyte count and the plasma HIV RNA level (viral load), are particularly useful as they are highly predictive of outcome.

It is important to remember that some levels, such as CD4 lymphocyte numbers, can vary significantly according to a number of factors including the time of the day the sample is taken and if other infection is present. Therefore, care must be taken in interpreting results and serial CD4 lymphocyte testing is likely to give a more accurate picture of disease progression.

Medical treatment strategies for HIV infection have been described in three main categories (Weller and Williams 2001):

- Antiretroviral therapy to suppress viral replication that can lead to improved immune function and longer life expectancy
- Prophylactic treatment against opportunistic infections
- Prevention of exposure to opportunistic pathogens.

Such medical strategies have to be considered alongside many other psychosocial factors in an individual's life, including their response and adaptation to their diagnosis, levels of social support, and general health issues such as diet. These factors, and many others, interweave to affect how an infected individual responds to the medical treatment strategies that can be offered.

Antiretroviral therapy

Following the introduction of highly active antiretroviral therapy (HAART) in 1996 HIV infection can be managed as a chronic infection, and the predicted life span for an individual has increased. The use of HAART has led to a significant decline in the incidence of new cases of AIDS and AIDS associated deaths (Weller and Williams 2001).

How HAART works

There are four main groups of antiretroviral drugs:

● Nucleoside analogue reverse transcriptase inhibitors (NRTIs)
● Non-nucleoside reverse transcriptase inhibitors (NNRTIs)
● Protease inhibitors (PIs)
● Nucleotide analogue reverse transcriptase inhibitors (NtRTIs).

For an illustration of antiretroviral therapy see Figure 3.1.

Table 3.2 Licensed antiretroviral drugs for adults with HIV infection

Nucleoside Analogue Reverse Transcriptase Inhibitors	Non-nucleoside Reverse Transcriptase Inhibitors	Protease Inhibitors	Nucleotide Analogue Reverse Transcriptase Inhibitors
AZT/Zidovudine	Nevirapine	Indinavir	Tenofovir
ddI/Didanosine	Efavirenz	Ritonavir	
ddC/Zalcitabine	Delavirdine	Saquinavir	
d4T/Stavudine		Nelfinavir	
3TC/Lamivudine		Amprenavir	
ABC/Abacavir		Lopinavir/Ritonavir	
AZT+3TC combined Combivir			
AZT+3TC +Abacavir combined Trizivir			

Figure 3.1   Antiretroviral therapy

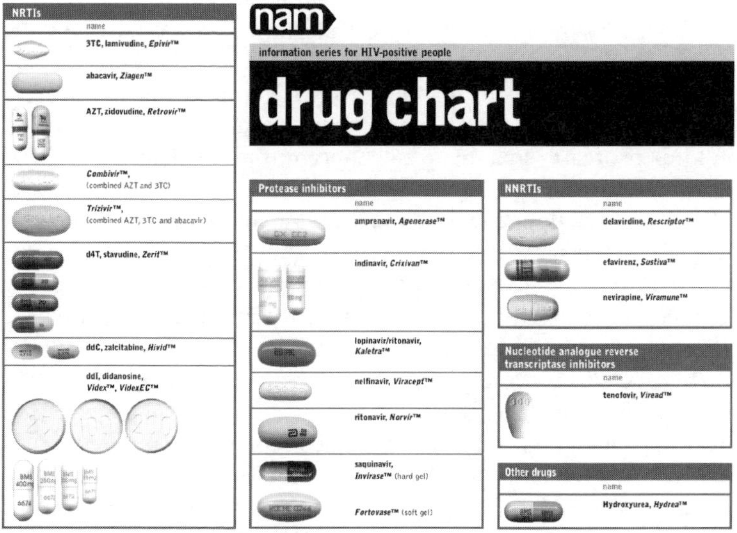

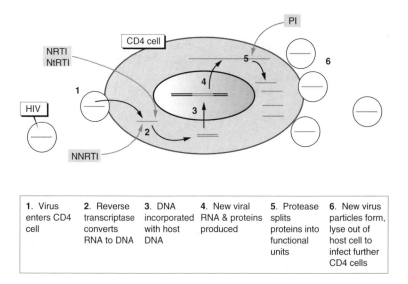

Used with permission from NAM

Figure 3.2   Life cycle of HIV and drug site of action

1. Virus enters CD4 cell	2. Reverse transcriptase converts RNA to DNA	3. DNA incorporated with host DNA	4. New viral RNA & proteins produced	5. Protease splits proteins into functional units	6. New virus particles form, lyse out of host cell to infect further CD4 cells

The first two groups, nucleoside analogue reverse transcriptase inhibitors (NRTIs) and non-nucleoside reverse transcriptase inhibitors (NNRTIs), used initially in the early 1990s, affect the action of the HIV reverse transcriptase enzyme. This enzyme is a catalyst for the virus to become integrated into the host cell.

The third group, protease inhibitors (PIs), which came into clinical use in 1996 in the United Kingdom, act by inhibiting the action of the viral protease enzyme which is required to help other HIV proteins mature.

Nucleotide analogue reverse transcriptase inhibitors (NtRTIs) also affect the action of reverse transcriptase, and the drug Tenofovir was approved in the United Kingdom in February 2002. It is licensed for use in people who have used other antiretroviral drugs previously.

Figure 3.2 illustrates how antiretroviral drugs work.

When NNRTIs were used as single (mono) therapy, resistant strains of the virus emerged with subsequent loss of antiviral effect. The drugs therefore need to be combined (combination therapy) and HAART usually comprises three or more drugs, often two NRTIs with either one NNRTI or one or two PIs (Weller and Williams 2001, Kulasegaram and De Ruiter 2001). Studies have shown an association between the use of combination therapy, a reduction in viral load and improved clinical outcome, which includes an improvement in immune function (Weller and Williams 2001). Guidelines about the use of antiretroviral therapy have been developed (British HIV Association 2001).

Side effects

There are side effects associated with most antiviral treatments. Rashes are relatively common. In severe cases Stevens-Johnson syndrome has been reported, with some fatalities. Other side effects include:

- Fever
- Diarrhoea and vomiting
- Fatigue
- Headaches
- Liver dysfunction
- Metabolic disorders
- Mitochondrial toxicity including lactic acidosis and lipodystrophy.

Lactic acidosis (high lactate levels) is very rare but is a serious side effect of the nucleoside reverse transcriptase inhibitors. Lipodystrophy, abnormalities of body fat redistribution often accompanied by elevated lipids and impaired glucose tolerance, has been associated with patients receiving HAART (Aldeen 1999). This side effect can be particularly distressing for infected men and women as it can be a very visible sign of their illness and negatively affect their body image.

Men and women may report other side effects that they experience with HAART, and it is important for clinicians to investigate them appropriately as well as provide reassurance.

Drug interactions

With HAART it is essential to be aware of possible drug interactions if an individual is taking other medication.

Drugs such as antihistamines and the sedative agent midazolam in conjunction with protease inhibitors may cause higher levels of the former resulting in potential complications.

Similarly, some studies have indicated that levels of sildenafil (Viagra) have been shown to increase significantly in the presence of saquinavir and ritonavir, both protease inhibitors. Complementary medicines may also cause drug interactions; St John's wort reduces indinavir concentrations (Kulasegaram 2001).

When considering antiviral therapy for HIV infected drug users it is important to be aware of possible drug interactions, for example zidovudine (NRTI) and sodium valproate. In the case of ecstasy and ritonavir, fatalities have been reported (Brettle 2001).

Information about drug interactions and HAART is likely to change regularly and it is vital that clinicians and patients are alert to and informed about such a possibility (www.hiv-druginteractions.org).

Adherence

Essential to the effectiveness of these drug therapies is the patient's ability to tolerate and continue with the regime, also described as adherence. All antiretroviral therapies have to be taken every day, and it is important not to miss a dose as resistance to drugs may develop. All medications have to be taken at specific times, before, with, or after food, and some may involve other dietary instructions or certain food restrictions. This may be particularly difficult if an individual has not told any members of his or her family or friends of their diagnosis as they may then be questioned as to why they are taking medication. Therefore the involvement, motivation and personal circumstances of the individual play an equally important part in any decisions made about antiviral treatment.

Drug resistance

Infection that has a poor response rate to antiviral therapy may be due to resistant strains of the virus that have emerged. Resistance testing assays, which are described elsewhere, may provide useful information to help the clinician and patient to identify a different combination of antiviral therapy, either when commencing treatment or if the regimen is not effective (Weller and Williams 2001).

When to start highly active antiretroviral therapy (HAART)

In making a decision about when to commence antiretroviral therapy, a number of factors need to be considered. These include:

- The risk of disease progression including such indicators as CD4 count and viral load level. The British HIV Association (BHIVA) guidelines suggest that patients with a CD4 count of less than 200 cells/mm^3 and/or those with a high viral load of more than 30,000 copies/ml and patients with symptomatic HIV infection or AIDS should be offered HAART (British HIV Association 2001). If the individual declines to commence treatment, it is suggested that their viral load and CD4 count are monitored frequently (about every two to three months) and that the decision about treatment is also reviewed regularly.
- Commencing antiretroviral therapy can improve immune function so may be useful when an individual has an opportunistic infection (Weller and Williams 2001).
- As previously mentioned, there is also some debate about whether antiviral therapy would be effective following primary HIV infection, but the evidence is not clear.
- Whether the individual wishes to commence treatment. As adherence to any treatment regimen is vital, if an individual does not wish to commence treatment, those wishes should be respected.
- If the individual is considering having children, he or she may wish to delay treatment until after this time, but this may also depend on the clinical stage of disease. It is important to discuss this particular issue before starting treatment as, if pregnancy is being considered, this factor may affect which type of HAART is chosen. If pregnancy is not being considered then effective contraception, which does not interact with HAART, needs to be chosen.
- The choice of combination of antiretroviral drugs will be influenced by these factors as well as by professional guidance (BHIVA 2001).

Once therapy has been commenced the individual will need regular clinical monitoring and review to assess the effectiveness of treatment and possible side effects. If the viral load rebounds or if there are significant side effects, the regimen may need to be altered, though such decisions require careful consideration. There are concerns as to how long such therapy may be effective for, with the emergence of strains of the virus that are resistant to therapy, and this area is being researched. Individuals may require reassurance regarding this.

Prophylaxis against opportunistic infections

Equally important in the management of HIV infection is reducing the chance of opportunistic infections that may occur when the individual is immune compromised. If an individual's CD4 count falls below $200/10^6$ per litre the risk of such infections increases. Such infections include:

● Pneumocystis carinii pneumonia (PCP)
● Toxoplasma
● Cryptosporidium
● Cytomegalovirus
● Tuberculosis.

Pneumocystis carinii pneumonia (PCP)

Pneumocystis carinii is a fungal organism that does not appear to cause problems in healthy people, but in those that have a compromised immune system it can become a pathogen causing pneumonia. It is an important cause of death in patients with HIV/AIDS, but can also affect other immune compromised individuals such as patients with cancer, those on immunosuppressive medication following organ transplantation and premature infants (Bastow 2000).

Treatments include the following:

● Co-trimoxazole
● Pentamidine isethionate
● Atovaquone
● Trimetrexate
● Corticosteroids.

After an episode of treated PCP infection, maintenance therapy is necessary until the immune system improves and low dose co-trimoxazole daily is recommended in this situation. Additionally, prophylaxis for PCP is usually commenced when the CD4 count falls below $200/10^6$ per litre.

Similarly, the other infections mentioned (toxoplasma, cryptosporidium, cytomegalovirus and tuberculosis) may occur when an HIV positive individual is immune deficient. Guidelines for prophylaxis and/or treatment should be followed. It is important to remember that antiretroviral treatment helps improve immune function and that will also reduce an individual's susceptibility to opportunistic infection.

Exposure to opportunistic pathogens

Advice should also be available to individuals on how to reduce their risk of exposure to opportunistic pathogens. For example, to reduce their risk of infection with toxoplasma, individuals should be advised not to eat raw or undercooked meat and to avoid directly handling cat faeces.

Other pathogens may reactivate if there is immune deficiency, and appropriate advice and treatment should be given where possible.

Summary

- HIV is an incurable infection that causes progressive immune suppression that, in the absence of multi-antiretroviral therapy is associated with a very high mortality rate.
- However, in countries where HAART is available and there is appropriate management of opportunistic infections, the course of HIV disease has changed considerably in recent years leading to an improved prognosis. This has been described as the 'Lazarus effect' as the improvement in health has been so significant.
- Decisions relating to such therapy can be complex, and require clear two-way communications between those professionals involved and the infected individual.

Chapter 4

Transmission of HIV from mother to child

This chapter will explore the transmission of HIV from mother to child, also known as vertical transmission. This can occur during pregnancy, birth or while breast feeding. An understanding of vertical transmission, and what affects it, can assist in the implementation of strategies to reduce the rates of infection in children and optimise pregnancy outcome for infected women.

Timing of transmission

There is evidence that transmission of the virus can occur before birth and that the virus can cross the placental barrier. Early data came from the isolation of the virus from fetal material following miscarriage or termination of pregnancy (Lewis et al 1990). The virus has also been isolated in the genital tract and in breast milk.

Infants in whom HIV can be detected within 48 hours of birth are thought to have been infected in utero. Those in whom it is not detected at birth, but is present after 48 hours of age, and who are not breast fed, are considered to have acquired HIV around the time of delivery. It is believed that approximately 30-50% of vertical transmission occurs in utero and 50-70% at or around the time of birth (Kuhn et al 1997).

Whilst the exact mechanism of vertical transmission is not certain, chorioamnionitis, prolonged rupture of membranes, prematurity, intrauterine growth retardation and prolonged labour appear to play an important role in in utero transmission. Transmission during labour may be due to transplacental microtransfusion as placental integrity is disrupted, or may occur across mucous membranes or through breaches in the skin (Tudor-Williams and Lyall 1999).

Vertical transmission rates (VTR) have varied according to the population studied. Before the availability of interventions that have been shown to be effective these rates ranged between 15% and 45% (Mofenson 1994). With increasing knowledge of factors that affect vertical transmission, and uptake of particular interventions, in certain parts of the world including the United Kingdom, rates can be as low as 2% (Duong et al 1999).

Factors that may affect vertical transmission

There are a number of factors that have been shown to affect the rate of vertical transmission and these can be divided into five broad categories:

- Viral
- Maternal health
- Pregnancy and birth
- Use of antiviral therapy
- Type of infant feeding.

Viral factors

As previously stated, two variants of HIV have been identified: HIV 1 and HIV 2. Whilst in its natural course HIV 1 has a vertical transmission rate of 15-45%, the rate for HIV 2 infection is significantly lower, at 0-4%, and is rarely seen (Andreasson et al 1993). Different viral genotypes and phenotypes may also affect the transmission rate as well as the levels of HIV RNA (viral load).

The risk of perinatal transmission appears to be very low in women with undetectable plasma viral loads though transmission of infection has been reported at all levels of maternal viral load, and there appears to be no upper limit of viral load at which transmission always occurs (Anderson 2000, Ioannidis et al 2001). Viral load in genital secretions may also be important (Kovacs et al 2001).

Maternal health factors

The mother's stage of HIV infection as well as her general health can affect the rate of vertical transmission. Evidence from the European

Collaborative Study has shown that there is a higher risk for transmission if there is a low CD4 count, symptomatic disease or an AIDS defining illness. Additionally, women with primary HIV infection in pregnancy (that is, seroconversion) are also at increased risk for vertical transmission (European Collaborative Study 1996).

The presence of genital infections is a risk factor for vertical transmission of HIV. There is an association between infection with chlamydia, gonorrhoea or bacterial vaginosis and chorioamnionitis that, in itself, may lead to premature rupture of the membranes and/or premature birth. There is some evidence that the organisms associated with bacterial vaginosis may stimulate HIV expression. Additionally, where gonorrhoea and chlamydia have been treated in HIV positive women, levels of cervical mucosal shedding of HIV 1 RNA have reduced. Therefore such infections should be screened for and treated in HIV positive pregnant women (Lyall et al 2001).

If the mother has Hepatitis C infection, this may increase perinatal HIV transmission as well as the risk of vertical transmission of Hepatitis C (Manzini et al 1995, European Paediatric Hepatitis C Virus Network 2001). Lifestyle factors are also influential in relation to vertical transmission. Maternal vitamin A deficiency has been associated with an increased risk of transmission (Semba et al 1994) as has substance abuse (Landesman et al 1996), smoking, and unprotected sex with multiple partners (Anderson 2000).

Pregnancy and birth factors

In pregnancy, premature delivery at less than 34 weeks has been shown to increase the risk of vertical transmission (European Collaborative Study 1992, Kuhn 1997). The cause of the preterm labour, the immature immune system of the premature infant or genetic susceptibility may all contribute to such transmission (Anderson 2000) and, as previously mentioned, chorioamnionitis can also be influential.

Both prolonged rupture of membranes (for more than four hours) and premature rupture of membranes have been associated with increased vertical transmission (Landesman et al 1996). A meta-analysis from 15 prospective cohort studies, including over 7500 deliveries, stated:

the likelihood of transmission increased linearly with increasing duration of ruptured membranes with a 2% increase in risk for each hour increment. Women with clinical AIDS had the most pronounced increase in risk with a 31% probability of vertical transmission after 24 hours of ruptured membranes. (International Perinatal HIV Group 2001)

There has also been some suggestion that length of labour may increase the vertical transmission rate (Biggar 1996) and that amniocentesis and the use of invasive obstetric procedures such as the application of fetal scalp electrodes, fetal blood sampling, episiotomy or forceps may also contribute (European Collaborative Study 1992, Mandelbrot et al 1996, Anderson 2000) though others did not find any such association (Landesman et al 1996). There is also evidence of a higher risk of infection for the first born twin than for the second born (Goedert et al 1991). The use of vaginal cleansing does not appear to have any significant effect on vertical transmission except when the membranes had been ruptured for more than four hours before delivery (Biggar et al 1996).

An important consideration in birth factors that affect vertical transmission relates to the type of birth a woman has. A randomised clinical trial demonstrated that elective caesarean section significantly reduced the risk of mother to child transmission of HIV 1 without a notable increase in the risk of complications for the mother (European Mode of Delivery Collaboration 1999). Further support for the effectiveness of pre labour caesarean section came from a meta-analysis of 15 prospective cohort studies. The meta-analysis of 8533 mother-child pairs showed that the vertical transmission rate was 50% lower in women who underwent elective caesarean section before the onset of labour or rupture of membranes. This finding was independent of the effects of treatment with antiretroviral therapy (International Perinatal HIV Group 1999).

The techniques used during the elective caesarean section should aim to minimise contact of the fetus with maternal blood, and these include keeping the membranes intact for as long as possible, and washing the baby carefully on the table. Rapid clamping of the umbilical cord has been advised to avoid maternal-fetal transfusion during separation of the placenta (Johnstone 1996). A 'bloodless caesarean' method has been described that involves a vicryl stapling device for the lower segment incision and this can help minimise contact with maternal blood (Towers et al 1998).

There was concern that post-operative complications including wound infections are increased in HIV infected women, but the evidence was not conclusive, and complication rates appear to be related to the immune function status of the mother (Lyall et al 2001). As for all women undergoing caesarean section, antibiotic prophylaxis is recommended.

If the woman has an undetectable viral load prior to delivery there has been some debate whether a caesarean section, a procedure with its own risks, would still be beneficial.

Clearly when assessing risk for vertical transmission in an individual case there can be overlap between some of these factors such as premature labour, chorioamnionitis and premature rupture of the membranes, and it is important to consider them collectively rather than in isolation.

The use of antiviral therapy

One of the most significant factors to affect vertical transmission is the use of antiretroviral therapy for the mother and for the baby. The 076 study group carried out a randomised, double-blind, placebo-controlled trial on the safety and efficacy of zidovudine, where the drug (or placebo) was given in pregnancy, during birth and to the neonate. Results were initially available for 363 births that showed that maternal-infant HIV transmission was reduced by approximately two thirds, from 25% to 8% (Connor et al 1994).

Since this important finding, antiviral drug regimes, used with pregnant women, have developed further and mono- or combination therapy may be used. Decisions regarding what antiviral drug(s) to use and at what stage in pregnancy to commence them are complex. They are based on a number of factors that need to balance the health needs of the mother with those of the infant. Important points to consider include:

● Which antiretroviral drugs to use
● When to give antiretroviral drugs and how long for
● Drug resistance
● Side effects for the mother
● Side effects for the baby.

It is important to be aware that physiological changes in pregnancy may alter drug absorption, distribution, metabolism and elimination and so affect the drug dosing and side effects.

By early 2002, 16 different antiretroviral drugs were available, in the United Kingdom, for the treatment of HIV 1 infection, either licensed or on a named patient basis. These drugs are divided into the four groups, described in more detail elsewhere, of:

● Nucleoside analogue reverse transcriptase inhibitors (NRTIs)
● Non-nucleoside reverse transcriptase inhibitors (NNRTIs)

● Protease inhibitors (PIs)
● Nucleotide analogue reverse transcriptase inhibitors (NtRTIs).

Only the NRTI zidovudine is specifically indicated for use in pregnancy, though not in the first trimester, to reduce vertical transmission. For most other antiretroviral drugs prescription in pregnancy is cautioned and currently the only published studies are for monotherapy with zidovudine, nevirapine and ritonavir (Lyall et al 2001).

Monotherapy
In addition to the 076 study previously cited, studies involving shorter courses of zidovudine administration have also shown a reduction in vertical transmission (Shaffer et al 1999, Lallemant et al 2000). The development of viral resistance to zidovudine has only been found in small numbers of women at the time of delivery and has been associated with higher viral load and increased length of therapy. Limiting the use of zidovudine therapy to mothers with low viral load and high CD4 counts may lessen the chance of resistance developing (Lyall et al 2001).

The use of other NRTIs such as didanosine (ddI) and stavudine (d4T) as short courses in pregnancy is also being investigated.

Side effects of NRTIs may include headaches, fatigue, nausea, vomiting, rashes and blood disorders particularly in the first few weeks of treatment after which they often resolve. Rarely, they can cause mitochondrial dysfunction that may include peripheral neuropathy, pancreatitis, bone marrow suppression and lactic acidosis.

Early in 2001 agencies including the Unites States Food and Drug Administration advised that three pregnant women had died of lactic acidosis following treatment with stavudine and didanosine (two NRTIs) and that a further four cases had been reported (Food and Drug Administration 2001).

The NNRTI nevirapine has a rapid placental transfer and a long half life, and in the HIVNET 012 study, vertical transmission was reduced by 50% when two doses of nevirapine were given. In this study, women were given one dose of nevirapine in labour and the second dose was given to the infant between 48 and 72 hours of age (Guay et al 1999). However, resistance occurs frequently and rapidly when nevirapine is used as monotherapy both in the mother and in the infant (Lyall et al 2001) and therefore its use as single therapy is not recommended.

Side effects of NNRTIs can be similar to those of NRTIs but may also include rashes and liver problems such as biochemical hepatitis.

Rarely Stevens-Johnson syndrome may occur.

In the United Kingdom, monotherapy with zidovudine is recommended for pregnant women who do not need treatment for their own health as indicated by the CD4 count and the viral load measurement. Such therapy should be commenced before 32 weeks of pregnancy and the mother's therapy would stop after delivery (Lyall et al 2001).

Combination therapy

Guidance on the use of combination therapy in pregnancy is based on observational studies, some of which were small. Studies have assessed a variety of antiretroviral therapy combinations used in pregnancy including using two NRTIs (zidovudine and lamivudine) from 32 weeks, triple therapy including a protease inhibitor, and triple therapy including an NNRTI.

The Women and Infant Transmission Cohort Study (WITS) in the United States has indicated a reduction in vertical transmission to 1.1% in women taking antiretroviral therapy that included a protease inhibitor.

Though there has been some association between protease inhibitor use in pregnancy and preterm delivery, this does not appear to be conclusive (Anderson 2000, Lyall et al 2001, Tuomala et al 2002).

As well as the side effects (previously alluded to for NRTIs and NNRTIs) that may be seen when these drugs are used as part of combination therapy, there may be other effects from the protease inhibitors. These may vary amongst the different compounds but can include lipodystrophy, metabolic changes, kidney stones, hyperglycaemia and new onset diabetes. There is some evidence that women taking combination therapy that includes a protease inhibitor have a higher risk of developing diabetes mellitus during pregnancy (3.5%) than HIV negative women or HIV positive women taking either NRTIs or those who are on no therapy (1.35%) (Justman et al 1999).

The use of combination therapy in pregnancy is recommended when the woman's viral load is high, or her CD4 count is low and if she is already on combination therapy and becomes pregnant. In addition, if her viral load is not suppressed by the existing drug regime or she presents late in pregnancy or in labour, combination regimes for use both in the intrapartum and neonatal period would be recommended (Lyall et al 2001).

The results of resistance testing, described elsewhere, can also assist in determining the choice of therapy.

It is important to be aware of the possibility of drug interactions between antiviral therapies and any other medications administered in pregnancy.

For instance, concerns have been raised regarding increased metabolism of methadone (a drug used in addiction withdrawal programmes) when used with antiretrovirals including efavirenz and nevirapine – two NNRTIs. It is important for clinicians to be aware of such possibilities and to seek appropriate clinical and pharmacological advice when necessary.

Side effects for the baby

Information about adverse effects on the infant comes from a number of sources including animal toxicity studies, registry data, clinical trials and anecdotal experience. The possibility of adverse effects can be related to a number of factors including the drug itself, gestational age at exposure, the duration of exposure, the genetic make-up of the mother and the fetus and interactions with any other drugs to which the fetus is exposed.

There are national and international registers that collect such information including the Antiretroviral Pregnancy Registry, and the British Paediatric Surveillance Unit (BPSU), that follow up HIV positive and HIV negative children. The BPSU register links with the survey of HIV positive women in pregnancy in the United Kingdom carried out by the Royal College of Obstetricians and Gynaecologists. Data collected includes what antiviral therapy women have taken during pregnancy and birth. The BPSU recommend that infants who have been exposed to antiretroviral therapy should be followed up for at least five years. However, both these registers rely on voluntary reporting. Information regarding possible side effects is also available on line at www.hivatis.org.

Side effects of antiretroviral therapy in infants may be short- or long-term. The latter have been considered in four main groups: teratogenic, carcinogenic, developmental and mitochondrial. So far there has been no reported increase in levels of the first three groups (Lyall et al 2001).

Some cases of mitochondrial dysfunction in uninfected infants exposed to zidovudine were reported from France (Blanche et al 1999) though there was not felt to be a causal association (CEM/CMO/99/5). Also, some short-term side effects including symptomatic neonatal anaemia and abnormal liver function have been reported which appear to recover with supportive care (Lyall et al 2001).

Animal studies found efavirenz, a NNRTI, caused abnormalities in baby monkeys and this drug is not advised for use in pregnancy. In addition, there is some evidence that the risks of congenital malformation increase in those infants exposed in the first trimester to folate antagonists prescribed for Pneumocystis carinii pneumonia (PCP) prophylaxis and antiretroviral therapy (Richardson et al 2000, Jungmann et al 2001).

In summary, the use of antiviral therapy in pregnancy needs to balance the interests of the mother with the interests of the baby, but many advocate that treatment should be the same in pregnant and non-pregnant women (Anderson 2000, Kass et al 2000).

Guidelines have been produced which can help clinicians and women make informed decisions about the complexities of using antiviral therapy in pregnancy (Lyall et al 2001) which if used in conjunction with other interventions can help achieve reported vertical transmission rates of less than 2% (Mofenson 2001).

Knowledge about antiviral therapy is constantly changing and all clinicians need to keep abreast of the latest evidence regarding their use with childbearing women.

Method of feeding

HIV has been cultured from cell-free extracts of breast milk and infected cells have been identified (Thirry et al 1985, van de Perre et al 1993, Pillay et al 2001). Postnatal transmission of HIV can occur through breast feeding and women who are seroconverting are twice as likely to pass on the virus through breast milk as those who are chronically infected (Nicoll et al 1995).

Certain factors, such as cracked nipples and the duration of breast feeding, are considered to increase the risk of vertical transmission. An analysis of several studies showed that the risk of vertical transmission of HIV approximately doubles through breast feeding, giving an additional risk of 14% (Dunn et al 1992).

In a randomised clinical trial of 425 HIV 1 infected pregnant women, the effect of breast feeding and formula feeding on HIV transmission was assessed.

401 mother-infant pairs were included. The cumulative probability of HIV infection at 24 months in infants in the breast feeding arm was 36.7% compared with 20.5% in the formula feeding arm. The estimated rate of breast milk transmission was 16.2% although, because there was a lower compliance rate in the formula arm, this is likely to be an underestimate. In this trial, most breast milk transmission occurred early, by 6 months, and the use of breast milk

substitutes prevented 44% of infant infections and improved the rate of HIV 1 free survival at 2 years of age (Nduati et al 2000).

Follow-up of the women in this study indicated that maternal and infant survival may be further adversely affected by breast feeding compared to bottle feeding their babies. After 24 months, 10.5% of breast feeding women had died compared with 3.8% of bottle feeding women. Women who breast fed lost more weight than women who used formula feed, and weight loss was associated with an increased risk of death. Maternal death was associated with a 7.8 fold increase in the risk of subsequent infant death, even after controlling for the infant's HIV infection status (Nduati et al 2000a).

A further study carried out in South Africa indicated that exclusive breast feeding, rather than mixed feeding, reduces the risk of vertical transmission. 551 HIV positive women were counselled regarding the transmission risks associated with breast feeding and then self selected to breast feed or formula feed. Breast feeders were encouraged to practice exclusive breast feeding for 3-6 months. Mixed feeding was practised by 276/551(50%) of the sample. By 15 months the cumulative probability of HIV infection was higher in the mixed feeding group than in the exclusively breast feeding group (Coutsoudis et al 2001). However these data need to be interpreted carefully and further studies are required (Department of Health 2001b).

The World Health Organization (WHO), UNICEF and UNAIDS have endorsed recommendations on the prevention of mother to child transmission of HIV infection and infant feeding. Their collaborative statement reads:

When children born to women living with HIV can be ensured uninterrupted access to nutritionally adequate breast milk substitutes that are safely prepared and fed to them, they are at less risk of illness and death if they are not breast fed. However, when these conditions are not fulfilled, in particular in an environment where infectious diseases and malnutrition are the primary causes of death during infancy, artificial feeding substantially increases children's risk of illness and death. (World Health Organization 2000)

Thus exclusive breast feeding would be recommended in most resource poor countries if there were no access to safe breast milk substitutes either as a result of cost or hygiene considerations.

There is no evidence that if a mother is on antiviral therapy and breast feeding this will reduce the chance of HIV transmission to the baby (Lyall et al 2001).

In the United Kingdom, the Department of Health's policy is to advise HIV infected women not to breast feed in order to reduce the risk of transmission of HIV to their children (Department of Health 2001b) and this reflects current professional advice (Royal College of Midwives 1998, Royal College of Midwives and Department of Health 2000, Royal College of Obstetricians and Gynaecologists 1997). Women may require practical advice and support if the cost of formula milk and the equipment required for its safe administration is prohibitive.

If a woman chooses to breast feed, despite this professional advice, there has been some discussion as to whether this should be considered a child protection issue under the Children Act 1989 (Department of Health 2001b). This will be explored elsewhere.

Breast feeding can contribute to mother to baby transmission of HIV infection. It is important for those involved in maternity care to have a clear understanding of the issues relating to infant feeding in order to support HIV positive pregnant women in making an informed decision about how to feed their children.

Vertical transmission of HIV 2 infection

HIV 2 infection is much less common than HIV 1 infection, and vertical transmission rates are much lower in the natural course of disease at approximately 0-4% (Andreasson et al 1993, Smith et al 1998). There is no evidence to support interventions such as elective caesarean section, though antiviral therapy is indicated in pregnancy if the woman is symptomatic and CD4 cell count is less than 300 cells/mm^3 (Smith et al 2001).

It has been suggested that pregnant women with HIV 2 infection should be managed in a similar way to those infected with HIV 1 (Lyall et al 2001).

Summary

There are a number of interventions that can significantly reduce rates of vertical transmission of HIV infection. They include strategies aimed at:

● Decreasing maternal viral load and improving CD4 count by the use of antiviral therapy

- Decreasing viral exposure for the infant, including prolonged exposure to vaginal and cervical secretions, by the use of elective caesarean section
- Identification and treatment of risk factors such as reducing the risks of prematurity and treatment of sexually transmitted infections
- Reducing the risks associated with breast feeding by advocating formula feeding where possible.

All of these interventions need to be considered when planning and implementing care for HIV positive pregnant women. There is evidence that such strategies have been adopted in a number of countries and are acceptable to women (European Collaborative Study 1998, Lyall et al 1998) and that this has led to a significant reduction in vertical transmission rates.

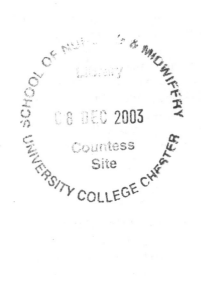

Chapter 5

Laboratory testing for HIV infection

There are a number of laboratory tests available for diagnosing and monitoring HIV and it is important to have a basic understanding of their use and relevance in HIV infection.

For those involved in providing screening programmes, awareness of the reliability and the limitations of the different assays available will help to give accurate information to those undergoing testing.

Colleagues in virology, immunology and other laboratory specialities are an essential part of multidisciplinary services for HIV infection, and are an important source of advice regarding the appropriateness and practicalities of tests and the interpretation of results.

Laboratory tests for HIV infection can be described in two main categories: the first group are used for screening and diagnosis, and the second for monitoring and management of patients once a diagnosis has been made. Issues regarding laboratory diagnosis of the neonate are also addressed.

Tests for screening and diagnosis of HIV infection

In routine screening programmes, such as those established for the antenatal population or for blood and organ donors, or as a diagnostic test for all but the newborn (infants up to the age of 18 months), HIV antibody testing is the method of choice. The limitations of HIV antibody testing for the newborn will be discussed later.

Figure 5.1 Laboratory testing

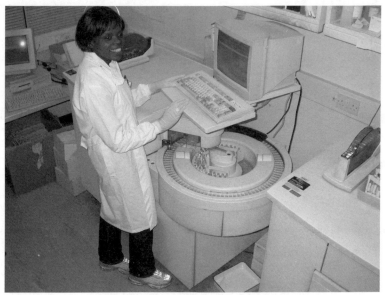

Used with permission of Lisa Brown, Medical Laboratory Assistant, Department of Infection – Virology section, Guys and St Thomas' Hospital Trust, London, United Kingdom.

HIV antibody testing – methods

Most HIV antibody testing is performed on serum but there are antibody assays available that utilise oral fluids. These have been used predominantly in surveillance surveys and in settings such as testing for insurance purposes. Tests have sensitivities and specificities in the range of 95-100% and 98-100% respectively (Lamey et al 1996).

However, testing using oral fluids is not commonly employed in diagnostic practice in the United Kingdom, where most testing is performed on serum, and this has been available since the early 1980s.

Commercial HIV antibody assays are cost effective in screening programmes, and many are now automated and can therefore provide a rapid 'turn around' time.

Three main types of assay are available: enzyme immunoassay (EIA), particle agglutination and Western blot (Lennette et al 1995).

Enzyme immunoassay

When testing by EIA, HIV antigen is attached to a solid phase and incubated with the serum. Captured antibody is then detected using an enzyme-labelled conjugate and substrate. Many assays detect antibodies to both HIV 1 and HIV 2. See Figure 5.2.

Figure 5.2 Detection of HIV antibodies by EIA

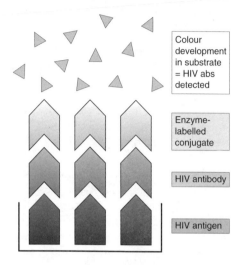

Colour development in substrate = HIV abs detected

Enzyme-labelled conjugate

HIV antibody

HIV antigen

Used with permission of Dr S O'Shea, Clinical Scientist, Department of Infection – Virology section, Guys and St Thomas' Hospital Trust, London, United Kingdom.

Figure 5.3 Detection of HIV antibodies by particle agglutination

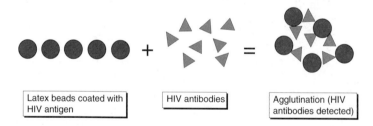

Latex beads coated with HIV antigen

HIV antibodies

Agglutination (HIV antibodies detected)

Used with permission of Dr S O'Shea, Clinical Scientist, Department of Infection – Virology section, Guys and St Thomas' Hospital Trust, London, United Kingdom.

Particle agglutination

Particle agglutination uses gelatin or latex particles, coated with HIV antigen, which are incubated with the patient's serum. Agglutination indicates the presence of HIV antibodies. A potential disadvantage of this type of test is that agglutination is read by eye so results can be subjective. See Figure 5.3.

Western blot

Western blot is used more commonly in the United States. When employed in the United Kingdom, it is used predominantly by reference laboratories. It identifies antibodies directed against individual polypeptides such as gp 120/41 and p24, which are coated onto nitrocellulose strips, which are then incubated with serum, enzyme-labelled conjugate and substrate. Coloured bands indicate the presence of specific antibodies.

All these methods are reliable with high levels of sensitivity and specificity. Low false positive or false negative rates are obtained and HIV testing is included in national, external, quality control schemes (NEQAS).

In the late 1990s, in a small number of cases, concerns were raised regarding the reliability of current HIV testing methods, specifically in relation to false positive results (Harrison and Corbett 1999). However, the cases referred to in this evaluation were all considered to have been related to failure to follow recognised diagnostic algorithms, possible misunderstanding of results by patients or mislabelling errors. (Chrystie 1999, Sheon et al 1994, Samson and King 1999).

HIV antibody testing – results

In interpreting antibody results it is important to remember that in the course of infection with HIV it may take up to three months for antibodies to develop. This period is called the sero-conversion or 'window' period.

Thus using an antibody assay alone may not detect those men or women whose infection is at this stage, and other molecular techniques will be required which are described later.

HIV antibody screening results are interpreted either as 'not detected', which is usually taken to indicate that the individual is not infected, or as a 'reactive' or 'antibodies detected' result that indicates infection with HIV. In some cases there will be an equivocal or discrepant result.

An algorithm for the interpretation of antibody screening results is shown in Figure 5.4.

Reactive results

With all reactive antibody results, a second sample of blood will be required in order to repeat the tests before confirmation.

In the United Kingdom, the assays normally used would be both antibody and particle agglutination.

Figure 5.4 Interpretation of antibody screening results

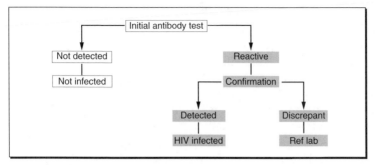

- *2 confirmatory assays/request for second serum
- Discrepant results could be due to; non specific reaction, early
  seroconversion, HIV-2 infection

Used with permission of Dr S O'Shea, Clinical Scientist, Department of Infection – Virology section,
Guys and St Thomas' Hospital Trust, London United Kingdom.

Figure 5.5 Interpretation of antibody screening results –
possible seroconversion

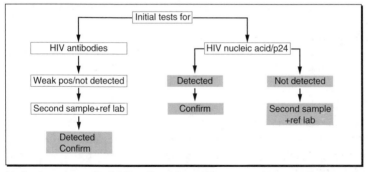

Used with permission of Dr S O'Shea, Clinical Scientist, Department of Infection – Virology section,
Guys and St Thomas' Hospital Trust, London United Kingdom.

The results of the tests on this second sample will either confirm
that HIV antibodies have been detected or demonstrate a discrepant
or equivocal result. Samples with discrepant results, or where the
result is weakly reactive, should be sent to a reference laboratory for
further, independent, analysis as well as testing a second sample.

Equivocal or discrepant results can be due to non-specific reaction
in the assay, early sero-conversion to HIV 1 infection or infection
with HIV 2.

An algorithm for interpretation of antibody screening results,
which may indicate a possible seroconversion, is shown in Figure 5.5

Testing for viral antigens/infectious virus

There are also assays and molecular techniques available that can test directly for viral antigens or infectious virus.

Detection of p24 antigen

P24 antigen is present at high levels in serum both early on and in the later stages of HIV disease. There are qualitative and quantitative assays available. In these methods, a solid phase is coated with anti-p24 antibody and serum, and enzyme conjugated with anti-p24 antibody and substrate is added.

Positive results should be confirmed by neutralisation.

It is important, however, to remember that p24 antigen is not always a consistent marker, and in current clinical practice, p24 antigen testing has been superseded, to a large extent, by measuring HIV viral load which is described later.

Detection of infectious virus

This involves co-culture of patient's peripheral blood mononuclear cells (PBMC) or plasma with mitogen-stimulated PBMC from an HIV seronegative donor, and monitoring cultures for production of p24 antigen.

It is a very labour intensive method and results may take up to a month, which is often an unacceptable length of time for clinicians and patients. In addition, a Category 3 containment laboratory is required. For these reasons isolation of HIV is mainly used as a research tool.

Molecular techniques

In the United Kingdom, molecular techniques, particularly for monitoring an individual's disease and their response to therapy, have been widely used since the mid-1990s.

However, the costs associated with such testing will prohibit their use in many resource poor countries.

Detection of HIV proviral DNA

For diagnosis of HIV infection, particularly during the 'window period' when antibody detection is unreliable, detection of HIV proviral DNA is a useful molecular technique. This highly sensitive method involves the use of PCR (polymerase chain reaction) to detect DNA in peripheral blood mononuclear cells.

HIV viral load (quantification of HIV RNA)

Viral load assays enable accurate determination of the amount of virus present in the blood. They measure the amount of cell free HIV RNA present in the plasma and the result is given as HIV RNA copy number per millilitre. The lower detection limit of most assays is 50 HIV RNA copies per millilitre.

The majority of tests for detection of HIV DNA/RNA were developed for use with HIV 1 subtype B, so their ability to detect non-B subtypes can be variable (Parekh et al 1999) which may result in falsely low or undetectable viral loads. In the United Kingdom, 78% of infections among women attending antenatal clinics are non B subtypes of HIV 1, with 61% being subtype A and 29% subtype C (Parry et al 2001). Therefore when interpreting results it is essential to have the full clinical picture, and if there are discrepancies it may be appropriate to retest using an alternative assay.

Measurement of HIV viral load is one of a number of baseline tests recommended for individuals following diagnosis. It should be measured regularly according to clinical criteria, to monitor disease progression and the patient's response to antiretroviral therapy. HIV viral load influences the rate of disease progression, and as a high viral load is associated with decreased survival time (Mellors et al 1996) the aim of treatment is to keep the viral load to undetectable levels.

Antiretroviral drug resistance

Antiretroviral drugs inhibit the activity of key enzymes involved in HIV replication, for example reverse transcriptase and protease. Drug resistance is mediated by mutations which alter these viral enzymes, thereby reducing or inhibiting their susceptibility to the drugs. Resistant virus can emerge rapidly when viral suppression is incomplete and antiretroviral drug resistance is a major cause of treatment failure, indicated by an increase in the HIV viral load.

Assays for detection of resistance to antiretroviral drugs are available and their value in therapeutic decision making is now well established.

These tests are based on either phenotyping or genotyping. Phenotyping involves culturing HIV from the patient's blood, in the presence of the drug, in order to obtain the inhibitory concentration. It may take a number of weeks to obtain a result. However, the turnaround time has been reduced by the development of high throughput automated phenotyping assays, based on recombinant DNA technology, which do not require HIV to be cultured directly from the patient. Genotyping uses PCR to amplify HIV from the patient's plasma. The HIV DNA is then sequenced automatically in order to identify mutations known to be associated with antiretroviral drug resistance.

Genotyping is generally used more widely than phenotyping as results can be obtained in a few days, rather than weeks, and the technique is technically less demanding.

Pregnant women on a non-suppressive antiretroviral regimen should have a resistance test conducted. Such tests should also be considered for antiretroviral drug naïve women, especially if there is an epidemiological risk of primary resistance, for example with an antiretroviral exposed partner (Lyall et al 2001).

Tests for monitoring and management of patients with HIV infection

Baseline tests recommended when an individual is diagnosed with HIV

HIV disease affects the immune system and can make the individual susceptible to opportunistic infections. Certain blood tests are recommended as a baseline following diagnosis in order to plan appropriate management. Some of these tests will be repeated at regular intervals during treatment in order to monitor the disease and its effects. Baseline tests include:

● Screening for Hepatitis B, Hepatitis C, cytomegalovirus, toxoplasmosis and syphilis
● Full blood count
● Liver function
● HIV viral load
● T cell enumeration.

T cell enumeration
This measures CD4 and CD8 ratio as a ratio and/or as an absolute cell number (x10^9/litre). The normal reference range for an adult CD4 lymphocyte count is 0.300-1.400 x10^9/litre though these reference ranges may be different in pregnancy.

Paediatric diagnosis

HIV antibody screening would be the method of choice for all paediatric diagnosis except in infants aged 18 months or younger.

Important issues of consent and other practicalities of testing with children are addressed elsewhere.

There are limitations to HIV antibody testing with the newborn. If antibodies are detected in this situation they may be maternal antibodies that have passively transferred across the placenta to the fetal circulation. Further antibody testing over the next eighteen months may indicate that the antibodies have declined, or a 'seroreversion' has occurred, and that the child is uninfected. Alternatively if the antibodies persist it could indicate a positive diagnosis for the child. Additional testing for HIV DNA and RNA, using molecular virology techniques, is used.

If by the age of 6 months HIV DNA/RNA are not detected the child is uninfected, although the child should still be followed up for 'seroreversion'.

If HIV DNA/RNA is detected and confirmed, and such confirmation can be given as early as 48 hours of age, then a positive diagnosis is made.

It may take up to 2-4 weeks for HIV DNA to be detected, and this can indicate whether the child was infected in utero or intrapartum.

Prior to the introduction of such techniques for paediatric diagnosis, it could often take many months before parents could be given a definitive result. However, testing infants for HIV DNA and RNA has enabled results to be given more quickly.

Summary

It is important for those involved in discussions with families about HIV infection to have a clear understanding of the different types of tests available and how results are interpreted.

- Serum antibody testing is the method of choice for screening programmes and diagnosis of infection in all but the newborn (<18 months of age).
- Antibody assays are reliable, with high levels of sensitivity and specificity, and false positive or negative results are rare.
- P24 antigen testing has largely been superseded by HIV viral load testing.
- Isolation of HIV is mainly used as a research tool as it is labour intensive, and results may take up to a month.
- Molecular techniques such as PCR (polymerase chain reaction) are now used widely in the United Kingdom for detection of HIV

nucleic acid (proviral DNA and cell free RNA).

● Detection of HIV proviral DNA is valuable for diagnosis during the 'window period' such as with seroconversion illness, or following needlestick injury, and in paediatric diagnosis when antibody detection is inconclusive.

● HIV viral load assays (quantification of HIV RNA)enable accurate determination of the amount of virus present in the blood.

● HIV viral load quantification is used to monitor disease progression and assess response to antiretroviral therapy.

● HIV viral resistance tests are a useful tool for clinicians in decisions about suitable treatment.

● Other essential tests for management and monitoring of HIV infection include full blood count, T cell function, liver function and other infection screening.

● Laboratory colleagues are an essential part of multidisciplinary services for HIV infection and should be referred to regarding the appropriateness and practicalities of tests and the interpretation of results.

Chapter 6

Testing for HIV infection for the childbearing woman

The aim of this chapter is to present an overview of the issues involved in testing for HIV infection, particularly for the childbearing woman.

As well as an awareness of the laboratory assays described elsewhere, an understanding of why testing is recommended and how to incorporate the routine offer into clinical practice is important for all involved in testing programmes.

In the early years of the epidemic in the United Kingdom, there was much debate on whether a test should be offered to every pregnant woman.

Was there a benefit for her and her baby, or was such testing solely to gain knowledge of the prevalence of the disease within the population?

Much has changed since that time both in terms of management of the disease, generally and in pregnancy, and in attitudes and approaches to the infection and testing for it. Testing is now more widely supported by professional and voluntary groups (Royal College of Midwives 1998, Intercollegiate Working Party 1998). In order to explore this further, HIV testing is examined under the following headings:

● Who may be recommended for an HIV test?
● When to test?

● Why test?
● How to offer an HIV test?

All these aspects of testing need to be considered by those involved in providing or developing a service.

Who may be recommended an HIV test?

Testing can occur in a number of settings. These can include:

Those presenting with symptoms of HIV infection

In the early years of the epidemic, men and women would be diagnosed with HIV infection as a result of presenting with symptoms of the disease. Common presentations included atypical pneumonias such as Pneumocystis carinii pneumonia (PCP).

The time from diagnosis of HIV to AIDS and then death could be relatively short, which made the issues around dealing with the illness particularly difficult.

With more widespread availability of testing, men and women can be diagnosed at an earlier, asymptomatic stage of the illness. This stage can be reflected in the individual's CD4 count at diagnosis, with a lower count indicating that a person's illness is further advanced. Reports show that the median CD4 count near to diagnosis was lower for those infected heterosexually than for those infected through sex between men throughout the 1990s. Guidelines for the management of HIV infected adults recommend that therapy is introduced before the CD4 count falls below 200 cells/mm^3 or 0.200 x 10^9/litre (British HIV Association 2001). However, diagnosis for more than half of heterosexually infected men and nearly half of the women is occurring after this stage of disease progression is reached (CDSC 2001).

Similarly, children would present with a variety of symptoms, including Pneumocystis carinii pneumonia (PCP), cytomegalovirus, encephalopathy or severe wasting, and the differential diagnosis would include HIV infection.

The majority of paediatric infection is via vertical (mother to baby) transmission. As well as the difficulties for the parents and the child in dealing with the latter's illness, for many parents there were additional concerns that one or both of them would be HIV positive too, and would therefore have to address their own diagnosis as well.

HIV infection and the neonate is explored further elsewhere.

However, both for adults and children, testing before having symptomatic disease can confer the advantage of having more time to adjust to the diagnosis, as well as to the appropriate introduction of antiviral therapy and other treatments.

Those felt to be 'at risk'

Testing can also occur if the individual identifies risk factors, and then refers him/herself for further advice. This may be to a service such as departments of sexual health, also known as genitourinary medicine (GUM) clinics.

In addition, risk factors may be identified by a clinician whom the individual is consulting regarding another health issue. Examples may include individuals presenting with other sexually transmitted infections including Hepatitis B, syphilis or gonorrhoea, or with other haematological disorders such as thrombocytopaenia. Such conditions can be associated with HIV infection but are not necessarily so.

However the assessment of risk 'is a shaky tool, an inexact probe for an inexact science' (Sherr 1991). The difficulty in categorising behaviours or people is that there will be over-inclusion of those who appear to have risk factors, and yet those who may be infected but who do not fit into any specific group may be missed.

For example, a survey of HIV positive women indicated that the majority of the sample, 81.3%, did not think they were at risk when they probably became infected, so would not have identified themselves as at high risk (Positively Women 1994).

The Department of Health has issued guidelines for pre-test discussion (Department of Health 1996). Factors which may need to be considered in any assessment of risk include:

- Unsafe sexual practice and its frequency for both partners. High-risk activity can include vaginal or anal intercourse without the use of condoms.
- History of drug use and especially injecting exposure.
- A history of exposure to blood or blood product transfusion particularly prior to screening of donations or heat treatment of Factor VIII, which was implemented in 1985 in the United Kingdom.
- Overseas travel with exposure to high-risk activity.
- Occupational risk.
- Tattooing (in any situation where single use sterile needles have not been used).

It is important to note that the assessment of risk, particularly in relation to issues of sexual health, may be sensitive and difficult to discuss with men or women in any setting. However, such discussions should be an integral part of maternity care as most women presenting for antenatal care have, by definition of being pregnant, had unprotected sex, and therefore have some level of risk for any sexual infection.

Testing as part of a wider screening procedure

Testing in pregnancy

The issue of testing pregnant women has been regularly, and often heatedly, debated ever since assays were developed (Goldberg and Johnstone 1993, Dunn et al 1995, Minkoff and Landesman 1998, Davies 2000).

The advantages and disadvantages of testing for this group of women at this stage in their lives have evoked strong opinions and feelings on both sides. However, as more information emerged about medical management of the disease and ways to reduce vertical transmission, so policy has altered.

Following UK Department of Health advice in 1992 and 1994 (Department of Health 1992, Department of Health 1994) the test was to be offered to all women in areas of high prevalence, and in areas of low prevalence, it was to be offered to women perceived by themselves, or their caregivers, to be at risk of infection. However, uptake was low, and this was partly due to national variation in testing policy.

For example, a survey in the mid-1990s showed that only 7% of units surveyed offered testing routinely, 21% selectively and 72% in response to client request (Ruby and Siney 1997).

The resulting detection rate of HIV infection in pregnancy was less than 20% (Nicoll et al 1998).

In the light of the medical and other benefits for the mother and child, of knowing whether or not she is HIV positive, the national guidance on antenatal testing was further strengthened.

The Department of Health issued recommendations for antenatal HIV testing policy in 1999 (Department of Health 1999). This followed advice from an Intercollegiate Working Party and is supported by voluntary groups (Intercollegiate Working Party 1998). A similar policy has been implemented in Wales and is being considered in Scotland and Northern Ireland.

In the Department of Health guidance there are targets to be achieved (see Box 6.1).

Box 6.1

All Health Authorities should ensure that arrangements are in place by 31 December 2000 at the latest:

● For all pregnant women to be offered and recommended an HIV test as an integral part of their antenatal care*

   *this does not include women arriving in labour or too late for antenatal care, who should be offered and recommended a test after delivery.

These arrangements should be designed to achieve:

● An increased uptake of antenatal HIV testing to a minimum of 50%

● For those health authorities that have effective monitoring systems in place and are already achieving an uptake of 50% or more, to increase uptake by a further 15%

All health authorities should ensure that arrangements are in place designed to achieve the following by 31 December 2002:

● An increase in uptake of antenatal HIV testing to 90%

● That nationally, 80% of HIV infected pregnant women are identified and offered advice and treatment during antenatal care.

It is anticipated that these targets will result in 80% reduction in the number of children with HIV acquired from an infected mother during pregnancy, birth or through breast feeding.

It is also recommended (Department of Health 1999) that this policy should be subject to monitoring and audit. Such monitoring should be able to provide information which includes the number of women who:

● booked for antenatal care
● were offered an HIV test
● decided to accept/decline a test (known as the uptake rate)
● were found to be infected (known as the identification or detection rate)
● accepted interventions to reduce vertical transmission, and which interventions were accepted.

Blood and organ donation

Since 1985, all donated blood and blood products are tested for HIV infection by testing the donor. In addition, blood products such as Factor VIII have been treated by heat inactivation methods since this time. All potential blood donors are asked to exclude themselves from donation if they have participated in any risk activities. If the test result of the donor is positive, the individual is either informed by being recalled to the Blood Transfusion Centre, or contacted via their General Practitioner, often in liaison with genitourinary medicine services.

Donors of any organs or tissues for human transplant are also tested, and if found positive, their organs would not be used. This principle also applies to breast milk banks where mothers are asked to self exclude if they are aware they are at risk for infections including HIV, and are tested for a number of blood borne infections including HIV (UK Association for Milk Banking).

Insurance

In certain circumstances an insurer may request an individual to have an HIV test before agreeing to provide life insurance. In this instance, individuals should be notified in writing of the need for an HIV test and the test procedure, and asked to provide their written consent and nominate a doctor to take the blood sample and receive the result. The pre-test discussion and post-test counselling will be arranged by the doctor.

There are other situations in which testing will be discussed and recommended, as it becomes more common and part of routine health care.

When to test

The early detection of HIV infection by antibody testing can confer a number of benefits. (Department of Health 1996)

These include allowing the individual to obtain medical and supportive health care, and to take action to prevent transmission. Early detection in women allows them to make informed decisions about conception and the management of pregnancy, including infant feeding.

Clearly, there is a place for pre-conceptual testing to allow couples to know prior to pregnancy if either is infected, and in certain parts of the world a pre-marital testing service is available. Pre-conceptual diagnosis may give either partner more time to deal with issues arising from results.

However, currently, many couples do not appear to access any formal pre-conceptual service, either in general practice, family planning clinics or other settings, so would not be diagnosed through this route.

Testing in assisted conception units and fertility services has become more widespread (Hart et al 2001). 42% of assisted conception units in the United Kingdom tested for HIV in 1999 (Marcus et al 2000).

However, as most women do not require such services in order to conceive, the opportunity for testing for the childbearing woman is most commonly addressed in pregnancy, generally at the first, or booking, appointment.

Recommendations for testing in pregnancy reflect the guidance that diagnosis should be at as early a stage as possible. This allows those diagnosed HIV positive the opportunity to be offered advice and treatment during antenatal care for their health and that of their baby (Department of Health 1999).

One of the concerns regarding policies which recommend testing for pregnant women as part of their antenatal care is whether pregnancy is the best time for a woman to find out she is HIV positive. Dealing with the many issues that can arise following such a result is obviously difficult in pregnancy, but deferral of diagnosis till a more appropriate time, whenever that might be, can bring its own problems.

If a woman is infected, she is likely to find out at some point, either through becoming ill herself or via the paediatric services. It has been said that an even worse time to find out you are HIV positive is when you have a sick child. The response of some women to diagnosis via paediatric services has been to express amazement to clinicians that they were not tested in pregnancy, when numerous bottles of blood are taken (Mercey and Nicholl 1998). Some women have talked of litigation in these circumstances.

Such experiences have influenced guidance about the importance of pregnancy as a time to have an HIV test.

The essential point to stress however is that whenever an individual is diagnosed with HIV, appropriate, supportive services need to be in place.

Why test?

Though HIV/AIDS has been described for 20 years, and there is evidence of its existence before that, it is still a relatively new disease. Information about its spread, transmission and the life expectancy of those with the illness is constantly changing.

In the early years, following the development of antibody screening tests, benefits to an individual in knowing whether or not they were HIV positive were felt to be less clear than they are now.

In clarifying a decision on the reasons for any screening test, a number of considerations should be addressed.

The National Screening Committee has proposed a new definition of screening, taking into account the importance of informed choice and risk reduction:

a public health service in which members of a defined population, who do not necessarily perceive they are at risk of, or are already affected by, a disease or its complications, are asked a question or offered a test to identify those individuals who are more likely to be helped than harmed by further tests or treatment to reduce the risk of disease or its complications. (Department of Health 2000b)

When testing is considered, the benefits and any harm, whether to the group or to the individual, must be clearly assessed and informed consent gained (Department of Health 2001).

Benefit to mother and child and reduction of vertical transmission

As early as 1992 it was recognised that there may be clinical benefits to the mother and her child of knowing their sero-status:

Evidence now suggests that an infected person may benefit clinically from prophylactic treatments to delay the onset of HIV related disease and from earlier treatment of any such conditions. Therefore testing for HIV infection can benefit both the individual and the public health. (Department of Health 1992)

One of the main arguments for named antenatal testing was, and is, that, if a positive diagnosis is made, the woman and, where possible, her partner would have time to consider options available to them and to plan their pregnancy care. Such options include:

● Access to treatment for the mother
● The availability of drug therapy to help reduce the chance of

vertical transmission
- Information about care in pregnancy, the most appropriate type of delivery and care after the birth
- Advice on infant feeding.

Knowledge of HIV status prior to delivery allows the mother to consider the use of antiviral therapy for herself and her baby, and to make an informed decision on the most appropriate type of birth. It has been shown that, if the mother labours, the use of invasive procedures, prolonged rupture of membranes and a long labour may all increase the chance of vertical transmission. There is also evidence that birth by elective caesarean section can reduce the chance of transmission. A full discussion of the use of antiviral therapy, and the advantages and disadvantages of both types of delivery, should be offered to allow a woman to make her informed choice.

The reduction of vertical transmission by avoidance of breast feeding is also an important factor in considering testing in the antenatal period.

Further examination of all of these issues occurs elsewhere.

There is evidence to suggest that women who are diagnosed HIV positive and are pregnant are increasingly taking up interventions which lead to a reduction in perinatal transmission (Duong et al 1999).

For most mothers, the most important consideration in pregnancy is to have a healthy baby (Larsson et al 1990, Laurent 1995) and they will accept such interventions to achieve this.

Termination of pregnancy, though not often taken as result of testing HIV positive, is an option for women (Johnstone et al 1990). There were concerns that women were pressurised into terminations (Massiah 1993). It is important that a decision about whether or not to continue with a pregnancy is taken in a fully informed and non-coercive manner.

In more recent years in the United Kingdom, many women choose not to opt for termination in the light of a number of factors. These include increased knowledge about the course of infection, reduced vertical transmission rates, as well as the social and cultural importance of motherhood for many women.

The option of continuing with the pregnancy when a woman is HIV positive, followed by adoption or fostering of the child can also be chosen, but obviously requires careful consideration.

Health promotion

Offering HIV testing can be used as an opportunity for health promotion.

When the health care worker discusses testing, it can provide an opportunity to inform women and their partners, if they are present, of the risks of transmission.

Such discussions can include information about risk behaviour, safer sexual practices and prevention of transmission. Safer drug using information can also be given.

A test, whether the result is positive or negative, can give the individual the opportunity to review their behaviour and change it if necessary.

Even if the individual declines the test, the pre-test discussion may effect change in behaviour. This factor is an important aspect to consider in antenatal testing, as if a woman is HIV negative, helping her to remain uninfected is the most effective way of reducing vertical transmission.

Epidemiology

The gaining of epidemiological data has also been cited as one of the benefits of testing for HIV. Such data on prevalence and spread within populations can assist in monitoring public health programmes and their effectiveness.

The antenatal population are one of a number of surveyed groups. They reflect a cross section of the population. The majority of them are heterosexual, and, by definition, have been sexually active.

In addition, the women all have blood taken for routine antenatal investigations, thus facilitating the collection of the samples.

For prevalence monitoring, anonymous, unattributable testing can be used.

The test result cannot be linked to the person, so information gained concerns the population tested rather than the individual.

Such prevalence surveys were introduced in 1990, and provide valuable statistical data to monitor patterns of the infection in the pregnant population.

They have shown that the antenatal population has a lower prevalence of HIV infection than other groups who undergo HIV testing such as homosexual, bisexual and heterosexual men and women who attend genitourinary medicine clinics, and injecting drug users (Department of Health 2000a).

However, anonymous, unlinked sero-surveys can present an ethical problem in that there may be unidentified individuals who are HIV positive, and cannot be informed of the result, as it is anonymous. The individual may be unaware of their status and may require treatment or care.

For this reason, when they were established, it was stated that alongside the anonymous unlinked programme there must be the facility for named, linked testing (Gill et al 1989).

It has been demonstrated that women have misunderstood this. In a survey of 222 pregnant women who had taken part in an anonymised, unlinked programme, 18 had had named testing discussed and 14 had chosen to be tested. Of the remaining 204 women, 84 (41%) believed they had had a named test, 64 (31%) said they had not been tested, and 56 (27.4%) were unsure. Of the 84 who believed they had had a named test, 76/84 (90%) believed the result had been negative and eight did not know their result (Desmond 1994).

Recommendations regarding named, attributable testing have been strengthened since this survey was carried out, and uptake of such testing increased, so that now more women are likely to be aware of their results. However, it is still important that women and health care workers understand the difference between named screening and anonymous unlinked surveys. The latter are for statistical purposes only.

Attributable testing, where the result can be linked to the individual by a number, initials, code or false name also occurs most commonly in the genitourinary medicine clinic setting.

Infection control

Infection control has sometimes been cited as a reason for testing.

In a survey of consumers' views on antenatal testing, one of the reasons given for the test being compulsory was 'to safeguard health professionals' (Meadows et al 1993a).

An assumption behind such reasoning is that if a health care worker knows someone is HIV positive they will adopt different, and presumably more stringent, infection control precautions.

However, if health care workers practice differently according to their knowledge of whether an individual is HIV negative or positive, their actions may reflect inaccurate assumptions.

As stated previously, a negative HIV result indicates no antibodies have been detected *at the point of testing* but the production of such antibodies can take up to three months.

Indeed if an individual is seroconverting, and does not yet have detectable antibodies in a serum sample, the blood is highly infectious at this time.

Thus, the practice of universal infection control precautions (UICP) is recommended, and is based on the assumption that all blood and certain body fluids of all patients are potentially infectious for any blood borne viruses, including HIV.

By managing all body fluids as if they were infectious, a health care worker is able to practice safely and in a non-discriminatory fashion.

An individual does not need to have an HIV test, and the health care worker does not need to know an individual's HIV result, in order to do this.

Therefore the practice of appropriate infection control measures by health care workers is not a reason for an individual to have a test.

The main reason for an individual to know about their HIV status is to enable them to make decisions in relation to their health and, in the context of pregnancy, the health of their unborn child. It is acknowledged that decisions about health are not made in isolation from an individual's social and cultural context and this needs to be considered as well when discussions about testing occur.

How to offer testing

Various factors need to be considered when examining antenatal HIV testing in order to be able to provide a service for women that is appropriate to their needs. These factors include:

- Training and knowledge of heath care workers about HIV infection, including a clear understanding of the process of testing.
- What consumers of the service think about testing, whether it is acceptable to them and that there is appropriate information for them.
- The provision of an easily accessible, multidisciplinary service for the care and support of HIV infected women.

All these factors should be regularly monitored in order to promote consistent standards nationally.

Training and knowledge of health care workers

A key requirement for the implementation of an antenatal HIV screening programme is training for staff involved. Their knowledge of the condition, including vertical transmission rates and the factors that affect it, and their ability to discuss this with pregnant women has been shown to affect uptake of the test (Gibb et al 1998).

Such training can also affect how midwives feel about their role in providing antenatal HIV testing.

In a study across three different maternity units, midwives without specific education and training were concerned about their lack of relevant knowledge and counselling skills to do the job. They also felt that 'ongoing education was important to achieve a sense of confidence in their knowledge and their skills in negotiating women's choice' (Roth et al 2001).

The role of other health care workers is also important. A survey of general practitioners' attitudes and beliefs on antenatal testing for HIV showed that although 84% believed that they should discuss the test preconceptually and during pregnancy, only 13% believed they always discussed the test antenatally. Knowledge varied, in that 88% knew that vertical transmission could be reduced, but 9% thought breast feeding should be actively encouraged. 48% believed that a negative HIV test would adversely affect life insurance (Whittet et al 2000) despite the statement, a number of years ago, from the Association of British Insurers, that 'a negative and routine antenatal HIV test will not affect applications for life insurance' (Association of British Insurers 1994).

It is important that appropriate training for staff is available in order that accurate, up to date information is given to women when discussing testing.

Such training needs to address not only knowledge but also attitudes to HIV infection and testing. Such attitudes may be linked to feelings about raising issues relating to sexual behaviour and sexual health within the maternity setting, as highlighted in Grellier's study (Grellier et al 1996).

It has been shown that the attitude of the health care worker to testing affects uptake more than their knowledge (Boyd et al 1999a). In this study, the midwife with the most positive attitude towards HIV testing caused women least anxiety, and achieved a higher uptake of the test. Other factors which may influence the uptake of testing are the age, experience and ethnic group of individual midwives (Jones et al 1998, Meadows et al 1990). Some of these factors have been highlighted in the presentation of other screening tests (Marteau et al 1992).

Training and education need to be ongoing to assist health care workers to keep abreast of changes in this constantly developing field and keep their practice up to date. In a survey of midwives' attitudes and practices regarding HIV testing, including integration of testing into routine antenatal care, midwives who had had more recent training had more positive attitudes towards antenatal HIV testing and care of HIV infected pregnant women (Low et al 2001).

Health care workers need to have access to clear written protocols regarding testing for HIV infection as part of routine antenatal care.

Such protocols should include practice regarding antenatal screening:

● Information about all antenatal blood tests should be included in one 'user friendly' leaflet, and in appropriate languages where necessary. This should be given or posted to the woman prior to her first appointment to allow her the opportunity to read it. This is good practice for any screening programme. However, such leaflets are designed as an addition to pre-test discussion, not as a replacement for it (Sherr and Hedge 1990). Health information needs to be available in other formats such as audio or video tapes for women who are unable to read or do not have English as their first language.

● A discussion should take place with the woman during the antenatal consultation or booking visit, about all recommended blood tests, and obtaining verbal consent for all of them from her. In some areas the use of a single blood test request form, with all appropriate tests included, has facilitated this process as well as reducing the amount of form filling for the health care worker. Although there have been concerns as to whether verbal consent is adequate for such testing, practitioners should be aware that 'a signature (of the woman) on a consent form does not itself prove the consent is valid – the point of the form is to record the patient's decision and also, increasingly, the discussions that have taken place' (Department of Health 2001). The signature of the health care worker on the request form for any screening, including infection screening or a fetal anomaly scan, implies that, following discussion, the woman has agreed. Such discussions and decisions about screening should also be documented appropriately in the woman's maternity records.

● The health care worker discussing antenatal screening needs to have an understanding of the process of the tests, including how long they take, and how the woman will be informed of negative or of positive results. In integrating HIV testing with other antenatal screening, it can be helpful to say that if there are any problems with the results of <u>any</u> of their antenatal tests, they will be contacted as per local arrangements. This may include being recalled by a phone call or by letter to discuss a result. Negative results may be given at the next antenatal appointment or, in some areas, with women's agreement, they have been sent by post (Smith 1996).

● Although all tests should be offered in a positive way, as a benefit for the mother and her child, it remains the woman's choice to accept or reject any of them, and she can have these tests at any time during pregnancy. Some units have adopted the policy of re-offering the HIV test at the 26 week antenatal check when repeat full blood counts are usually requested.

Thus, any person undergoing an HIV test should receive appropriate discussion prior to testing, so that they can decide whether to have a test in a properly informed way (Department of Health 1996).

This is important for all screening tests, including those recommended in pregnancy, as the conditions detected may affect many aspects of a person's life. Health care workers may find the use of a prompt card, with key points to include when discussing screening, helpful as an 'aide memoire' (Smith et al 1995).

Such a prompt card for discussion prior to antenatal screening tests should include information on:

● What conditions the tests are being recommended for, how they are transmitted (or may affect the woman) and why we routinely recommend testing for all women during pregnancy.
● Any interventions available to reduce significantly the effects on their own health and that of their child, including transmission to the baby.
● The benefits to them and to their baby of knowing these test results, whether positive or negative, and possible disadvantages.
● The tests, what they look for, how long they take and how the woman will be informed of her results.
● How to reduce transmission, particularly in relation to blood borne infection screening (that is for syphilis, Hepatitis B and HIV, which are the most commonly tested for infections in pregnancy in the United Kingdom). Guidance on safer sex, condom use, and safer drug use may minimise further risk to themselves or others. Such advice can apply whether the individual actually has the test or not. It is important not to take the individual's knowledge about blood borne infections and risk behaviour for granted. The risk factors

may need exploring. It is equally important not to worry the individual unnecessarily; risk behaviour does not automatically indicate the presence of infection.

● The confidentiality of these discussions. Whilst all information given in the course of a professional relationship has a requirement of confidentiality attached to it (UKCC 1992), women may benefit from specific assurances in relation to their sexual or drug using behaviour.

What do pregnant women think about antenatal HIV testing?

Studies have indicated that pregnant women think the test is important and acceptable (Meadows 1993a, Duffy et al 1998, Simpson et al 1998a).

However, having a positive attitude to a test does not automatically mean that a woman will accept it (Sherr et al 1996). As alluded to earlier in the chapter, the discussion with the health care worker is very influential.

Other influences which have been shown to be independent predictors of intention to be tested include benefit to the woman herself or her partner, being in favour of testing, being single, being younger, her perceived risk of HIV and knowledge that HIV can be transmitted by breast feeding (Meadows 1993b, Simpson et al 1998b). Indeed in Simpson's study the most frequently reported reasons for taking or not taking the HIV test were, respectively: 'It's a good idea to have it as a routine test' and 'I've been in a stable relationship for a long time' (Simpson et al 1998b).

Some reports indicate that there can be differences in the uptake of antenatal tests, according to race and ethnicity, where ethnic minority women were less likely to choose to have such tests (Kupperman et al 1996). In a survey of London maternity units, uptake of HIV testing varied by ethnic group from 9% to 24% (Gibb et al 1998). Similarly a study by Jean Meadows showed that women of Mediterranean origin were more likely to accept the HIV test than women from other ethnic minority groups (Meadows 1994). However a later study highlighted that neither ethnicity nor risk were predictors of HIV testing intention (Sherr et al 1998/9).

Partners can be an important influence in a woman's decision to test for HIV in pregnancy and can also affect women's experience of the testing process and whether they feel supported or unsupported in their decision (Baxter and Bennett 2000). Discussing support can raise issues of social and gender power relationships for the couple, which need to be considered when discussing sexual health in pregnancy. It has been suggested that it may be more beneficial to address such issues by counselling and HIV testing couples during pregnancy, rather than only women (Bott 2000).

As previously mentioned, since HIV testing has been available there has been concern about how pregnant women would feel about having the test. In an early study in 1988, whilst 82% of women felt the test should be available in antenatal clinics, only 48% reported that they themselves would take the test. At that time, anxiety levels surrounding the HIV test were significantly higher than for other routine antenatal tests (Stevens et al 1989). However, a more recent study has shown that anxiety was not raised where the test was offered to all, and where the midwife offering it had a positive attitude to testing (Simpson et al 1998a). Such findings reflect the changes in attitudes and approaches to HIV testing since the 1980s.

In-depth interviews with women about testing revealed that they felt some anxiety whilst waiting for results, but felt it was no worse than waiting for any other result. However, the way results were given caused considerable discussion, and it was suggested that this area may require further investigation (Boyd et al 1999b).

In summary, HIV testing programmes need to be sensitive to the views and experiences of women undergoing testing, who generally see the test as an acceptable and important part of antenatal care. Where health care workers are informed, up to date and have a positive attitude towards such screening, they will make a significant contribution to helping women to decide about testing and to deal with their results.

Results and post-test counselling

When a woman has consented to have antenatal tests, she should have been informed of when and how she will receive the results. It is important that a clear system is in place, otherwise she may (wrongly) assume that 'no news is good news'. Anecdotal examples exist of women who assume that if they have not heard anything, then all test results must be normal, whereas in reality the test may have been omitted, or the abnormal result not acted upon due to oversight or error. Some of these issues are illustrated in the personal perspectives on HIV testing in this book (see Chapter 9).

Each person undergoing a test should receive his or her result with post-test information and counselling. It is good practice for test results to be given in person.

A negative result

As previously stated it is important to inform the woman of the results of all her tests, including when the results are negative or show no abnormalities, as they are likely to provide reassurance and relief for her. She may have been particularly anxious whilst waiting for them. Most negative HIV results are given alongside the results of other antenatal screening tests.

Discussion and counselling following a negative HIV result should include information about the 'window period'. If it is three months or more since the last possible exposure to HIV, there is more certainty about the result. If there are concerns about recent infection, repeat testing at an appropriate time would be advised, as well as information on prevention. The possibility of further exposure should be explained, and the individual given the information to enable him or her to make choices about future safe behaviour.

It is important to inform the woman that her negative result does not automatically indicate that her partner is negative. The most reliable way for him to know is to have his own blood test, and some centres offer this.

It is important to use this opportunity to encourage behaviour change where appropriate, and to ensure that the individual, as well as being relieved, realises the limitations of a negative result.

A small number of women will remain anxious following a negative result, despite the apparent absence of ongoing risk factors for infection. They have been termed the 'worried well' and may need additional counselling and referral to specialist services for further support.

A positive result

Counselling following a positive result should be given in an appropriate setting with the relevant people available for support. This may vary according to local availability of staff, but may include a specialist counsellor or health advisor and a midwife or obstetrician. Obviously, it is important not to overwhelm the woman with too many staff.

Centres offering testing have developed protocols for giving positive results. Such results are rarely given on a Friday, when there are few agencies available over the weekend to give support. However, if there is a good support network of family, the weekend may be appropriate, with useful time off available for coming to terms with the result.

As with the giving of any difficult news, reactions will vary from individual to individual. It is important to allow time for the person to absorb the information; and, wherever possible, not giving such results in the middle of a rushed antenatal clinic, but arranging the appointment at the end of the clinic or another more suitable time.

It can be a very tense time. An individual's reaction to a diagnosis of HIV infection has been compared to the responses to death and dying described by Elisabeth Kubler-Ross (Forstein 1984). She describes four stages in receiving bad news: initially shock, then numbness and disbelief, next denial and finally acceptance. Whilst an individual may not rigidly adhere to this pattern, it is important for health care workers involved in giving bad news to be aware of likely responses.

Breaking bad news requires great sensitivity. People remember very clearly the way in which such information is given to them, and may go over it repeatedly through the rest of their lives. If it is broken clumsily, the individual's distress can be greatly magnified (Ashurst and Hall 1989).

In the context of a positive HIV diagnosis, there is often a desire for factual information about the illness, prognosis and treatment. There may be a need for repetition of information, as shock can often block comprehension. Response to the news will vary and depend on many physical and psychological factors. A strategy for care and management needs to be agreed with the individual, which includes a plan for those whom he or she can involve and turn to for support.

The checklist shown in Box 6.2 has been devised for use in HIV post-test counselling (Miller et al 1993). It gives a clear guide to the issues to be covered when giving a positive result in pregnancy.

Such guidance can be of great assistance to the health care worker in providing some structure to giving difficult news. For the patient, in this case the pregnant woman, hearing such news in a safe and contained way may help 're-engage her after the shock of diagnosis' (Miller et al 1993).

To be diagnosed whilst pregnant, and to have to consider the implications of having a life-threatening infection and the significance this holds for her child and her family, requires multiple levels of support for the woman at this time in her life.

The care and help for a woman with HIV infection in pregnancy is explored further elsewhere.

Box 6.2

- Recommend counsellor or specialist to be involved.

- Consider privacy of venue and time of appointment.

- Give the woman her result.

- Allow time for information to be considered and check what she understands by the result.

- Identify immediate concerns – common responses include 'Am I going to die?' ' What about my partner?' ' What about my baby?' ' How long have I had it?' Answer such questions as honestly as possible.

- Discuss whom the patient might tell about the result.

- Discuss what the patient might tell others and how they might tell others – role playing such a scenario can be helpful.

- Discuss how she plans to spend the next few hours and days.

- Identify what difficulties she foresees and how she might deal with them.

- Help her identify who else she might turn to for support.

- Encourage her to ask questions.

- Discuss health maintaining behaviours such as safer sex, good diet, sleep, exercise, etc.

- Assure the patient that the reaction of shock, anger or disbelief is quite common.

- Discuss specialist medical follow-up procedures and the benefit of prompt identification and treatment of symptoms.

- Give information about local support organisations.

- Always offer a follow-up appointment.

An equivocal result

On rare occasions a woman may receive an equivocal result. This may indicate that there has been a non-specific reaction with the HIV antibody assay, the early stages of seroconversion or HIV 2 infection. Counselling about such a result involves the giving of this information and the possible options. These include repeating the test, both locally and in a reference laboratory and using different assays as described elsewhere. Discussions should also occur about partner testing as, if the woman is seroconverting, there is a strong possibility that her partner will be positive, and will require treatment himself.

The client will need considerable support in this time to cope with the stress that this delay and uncertainty is likely to cause. Being unable to give a confirmed result for a number of weeks can cause significant anxiety.

Information about protection from further exposure from, and transmission to, others during this period must also be given.

Documentation, confidentiality and disclosure

Documentation

Professional practice guidelines for health care workers state that record keeping is an integral part of practice (UKCC 1998).

The issue of documentation regarding discussions and decisions about HIV testing and about results has been contentious, and has raised a number of questions. Should anything be recorded at all, or should there be a code to record it discreetly? If so, should this information be written in the client-held maternity notes, or solely in the back-up files kept at the hospital?

The practice of client-held maternity records is widespread in the United Kingdom, and has been valued for promoting good communications between the woman and all those involved in her maternity care. Particularly when antenatal HIV testing was less common than it is now, concerns were raised that, by documenting details of a decision regarding testing in such records, (which may be seen by other family members or friends) the woman would be stigmatised, even for having had the discussion. If the General Practitioner became aware that a woman had had a test, might this negatively affect a future application for life insurance or an endowment policy? This particular barrier to testing was addressed in

1994 when the British Association of Insurers issued a statement. This confirmed that applicants for life insurance proposals would no longer be asked whether they had had a test or counselling for HIV, but any question would be confined to asking only about positive test results or treatment (in line with other illnesses) (Association of British Insurers 1994).

However if there is no documentation of any action, such as discussing testing, or whether it was accepted or declined, there is no evidence whether or not such actions took place. That could raise medico-legal problems in the future. In addition, if the woman is seen by a different member of the clinical team, some documentation is important in order to ensure that she is informed of any results if appropriate and receives further support if necessary.

As HIV testing has become part of mainstream antenatal care, it is believed that the stigma associated with testing has reduced. Any discussions and actions should be documented in the same way as other sexual infection screening in pregnancy, such as syphilis or Hepatitis B. Thus, the treatment of HIV negative results should become one of a number of such test results that the woman receives, and which is documented appropriately in her maternity records.

All health care workers, in whatever setting, receive professional guidance relating to confidentiality of all health information, and they are required to adhere to it.

The Code of Professional Conduct drawn up by the United Kingdom Central Council for Nursing, Midwifery and Health Visiting (UKCC) states:

> As a registered nurse, midwife or health visitor, you are personally accountable for your practice, and, in the exercise of your professional accountability, must: ... protect all confidential information concerning patients and clients obtained in the course of professional practice, and make disclosures only with consent... (UKCC 1992)

Where people have suffered from breaches of confidentiality within health care settings, such conduct is subject to professional disciplinary proceedings, and civil action (UKCC 1992, UKCC 1996).

Documentation of positive result

The woman's positive HIV result should be documented in her genitourinary medicine records or hospital records according to local practice in order to facilitate ongoing care. Information in GUM records has additional confidentiality as provided by Section 2 of the

NHS Venereal Disease Regulations 1974. These state that:

> *any information capable of identifying an individual ... with respect to persons examined or treated for any sexually transmitted disease shall not be disclosed except: a) for the purpose of communicating that information to a medical practitioner in connection with the treatment of persons suffering from such disease or the prevention of the spread and b) for the purpose of such treatment or prevention.*

An HIV positive pregnant woman will have the standard 'hand-held' maternity record. Discussing with her what would be appropriate to document in her maternity notes, regarding her diagnosis, and her plans for treatment for herself and her baby is essential, so that she can have some control over such information. These discussions should clarify issues about disclosure, on a 'need to know' basis, to health care workers directly involved in her care, and the benefits to her of having key personnel aware of the situation. A small, multidisciplinary team can help facilitate this process, whilst ensuring that the woman does not feel that 'everyone knows'.

If such information is only disclosed verbally, or only to one person who may then be unavailable at the time of delivery, there is potential for treatment to be omitted, as the staff may not be aware it is required, and the woman may not feel able to inform them of her needs.

Some maternity units have found the use of a confidential birth plan, drawn up in discussion with the woman, to be helpful in addition to the woman's hand-held maternity records.

If the documentation is inappropriate, it may lead to inadvertent disclosure of the woman's status to family and friends if they have access to her hand-held records. This may have significant repercussions for her. In many countries, there is still a stigma attached to having HIV infection. For many people, there may be active discrimination, such as in employment or housing, if their HIV diagnosis is known. The social stigma can be considerable, with HIV positive individuals being shunned or rejected by their families, and subject to abuse.

The United Kingdom Declaration of the Rights of People with HIV and AIDS includes among its rights the right to privacy. It goes on to say:

> *We believe that information about the HIV status of any person should be confidential to that person and their appointed health and social carers ... Information should not be disclosed to a third party about a person's HIV status without that person's consent.*

A decision about disclosure to individual members of her family or friends is one that is taken by the woman with appropriate guidance from specialist services.

Summary

In conclusion, all health care workers involved in maternity care need to have a clear understanding of issues relating to testing for HIV infection for the childbearing woman.

- Testing has been shown to be acceptable to pregnant women as part of antenatal care.
- Midwives and others involved in maternity care need to keep updated on issues relating to HIV testing and pregnancy and to be able to discuss it, as part of antenatal screening, in an informed, positive and confident manner.
- Appropriate documentation should be made, balancing the requirements of professional practice and the needs of women in their care.
- Health care workers need to be familiar with the local arrangements for the care and support for women who are HIV positive and pregnant.

Chapter 7

Care during pregnancy, birth and the postnatal period

This chapter will explore various aspects of care that need to be considered for a woman who is infected with HIV and pregnant.

The underlying goal of care is to have a mother with optimal health and an uninfected baby. However it is not only physical health that is important but also psychological health, including the mother's response to her diagnosis, and an understanding of her cultural background and social support network. All these factors interlink. Care needs to be multidisciplinary in nature, with the woman and her baby at the centre of it. See Figure 7.1.

HIV positive pregnant women may have diverse needs. Whilst some will have been diagnosed before pregnancy, others will be informed of their infection as a result of a routine antenatal screening test, and their needs are likely to be different. It is important that services are flexible and sensitive to these varying requirements.

Aspects of pregnancy care can be examined from a number of perspectives though there is considerable overlap between them:

- HIV care following diagnosis
- Pregnancy care, the birth and the postnatal period
- Psychological health, counselling and support
- Disclosure, confidentiality and documentation
- Preconceptual care.

Figure 7.1 Multidisciplinary care

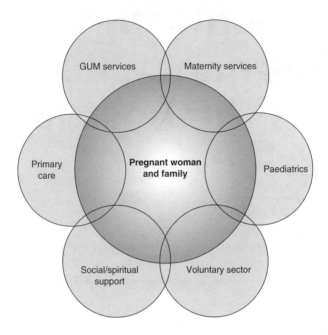

HIV care following diagnosis

Following diagnosis, the woman should be offered referral to specialist health services in order to monitor her HIV infection. In the United Kingdom, these are provided mainly within the acute or hospital-based setting, and this is usually situated within genitourinary medicine (GUM) clinics. Clinic personnel are likely to include medical and nursing staff and health advisors, as well as significant support from pharmacists, laboratory staff, dietitians and a number of community-based colleagues.

The woman may have concerns about what to expect when attending the GUM clinic, particularly for the first time, and a clear explanation of what is likely to happen at that first visit, such as multiple blood tests or other investigations or discussions regarding treatment, may help reduce her anxiety.

Baseline tests should include assessment of viral load, including resistance testing, CD4 lymphocyte enumeration, as well as screening for genital infections. Options for antiviral therapy and treatment of any infections will be based on the results of such investigations, and other factors that are explored elsewhere. Ensuring that the woman understands the nature of such tests, when the results will be available, and what treatment of HIV infection will mean for her is a complex process, and one that is likely to develop further at each appointment. Whilst colleagues in the GUM department may take the lead in discussing antiviral therapy, it is important that staff based in the maternity services have a clear understanding of the issues in order to provide consistent advice and information to women.

Concern has been raised that pregnancy may accelerate the progression of a woman's HIV disease, and it is important to address any anxieties regarding this. Pregnancy, without HIV infection, is associated with a decline in CD4 cells and a relative decrease in cell mediated immunity. Similarly, CD4 cells are expected to decline during pregnancy in HIV infected women, with eventual return to baseline levels.

A systematic review of studies indicated that, in industrialised nations, there was no significant acceleration of HIV disease although women with low CD4 counts may develop opportunistic infections (French and Brocklehurst 1998, Bessinger et al 1998) and women need to be reassured about this.

These results may differ from those seen in resource poor parts of the world where pregnancy has been associated with more rapid disease progression and maternal mortality. Such differences may reflect other factors associated with poverty, such as poorer nutrition, a greater likelihood of advanced HIV disease at the time of pregnancy, or the effect of other infectious diseases.

Appointments with the GUM team may be relatively frequent during pregnancy, particularly if the woman is newly diagnosed, or if alterations to her antiviral therapy are required. Clear communications between all the professionals involved and the woman may help her adjust to her diagnosis at this time.

Care during pregnancy, birth and the postnatal period

As for all pregnant women, antenatal care for an HIV positive woman should, as far as possible, be evidence-based and of a high quality. It is important that in our concern about her HIV infection, we do not overlook the fundamentals of pregnancy care. Appropriate schedules of antenatal care should be used which prepare for a healthy pregnancy and birth, provide information for mothers about pregnancy, birth and infant care, monitor maternal and fetal wellbeing, and offer appropriate referral if complications occur.

Many centres have developed family clinics where professionals from a variety of services are present and able to see the woman on a given day. Such services may include midwifery, obstetrics, GUM, paediatrics, addiction specialists, voluntary groups and other agencies.

Such clinics have the advantage of reducing multiple appointments for the woman, as well as facilitating communications between the different disciplines involved. However, it is important that the woman does not feel overwhelmed by seeing too many specialists in one day which could lead to 'information overload' and confusion. Many clinics have recognised this, and arranged that, although different professionals may be present, the woman will not necessarily see all of them at every visit.

As part of her antenatal care, screening will have been recommended for other conditions including infection screening (rubella, syphilis and Hepatitis B), and discussed for genetic and chromosomal conditions such as haemoglobinopathies and Down's syndrome. If diagnostic testing, such as chorionic villus sampling or amniocentesis, is recommended as a result of a haemoglobinopathy or Down's syndrome screening result, women should be aware of the possible risk of HIV transmission with the procedure, although there is little data in this area. Administration of antiretroviral therapy to cover the procedure should be considered (Lyall et al 2001).

An association has been noted between HIV infection and adverse perinatal outcomes such as spontaneous abortion, preterm delivery (particularly if the woman has advanced disease), low birth weight, intrauterine growth retardation and chorioamnionitis. Additionally, in resource poor countries there is evidence of increased risk of stillbirth, perinatal mortality and infant mortality (Brocklehurst and French 1998).

Those involved in maternity care should be alert for signs of such conditions, arrange for appropriate tests, and act on the results. For example, a link has been demonstrated between bacterial vaginosis and premature delivery, so it is good practice to screen HIV positive pregnant women for this condition, and treat where necessary (Lyall et al 2001). Women may also be susceptible to infections such as Candida albicans, particularly if they are immune suppressed, so careful monitoring is required. Monitoring fetal growth is essential in all pregnancies and, if there is concern, assessment by ultrasound should be arranged. The use of protease inhibitors as part of antiviral therapy has been associated with a higher risk of developing pregnancy-related diabetes, and this should be screened for as appropriate.

Dietary and nutrition advice and support is particularly important as women may have nutritional deficiencies such as anaemia or certain dietary requirements associated with their antiviral therapy regimes. An association has been shown between vitamin A deficiency and vertical transmission (Semba et al 1994). HIV positive pregnant women may require referral to a dietitian for further advice about their nutritional needs (NAM 2000).

If an HIV positive pregnant woman also misuses drugs, her needs may be even more complex. Her care will need to address the management of her addiction, her pregnancy and her HIV infection (and sometimes Hepatitis B and/or C) simultaneously. There may be difficulties with adherence to complex antiviral regimes, as well as the practicalities of phlebotomy in order to assess viral load, if there is poor venous access. Risks of preterm labour and delivery and intrauterine growth retardation associated with drug use may compound risks associated with HIV infection. It is important to have good lines of communication between the woman and all the agencies involved in order provide optimal care (Siney 1999).

There may be particular challenges in the prescription of antiviral therapy that may interact with recreational drug therapy. For instance, zidovudine levels are increased by opiates, whereas the absorption of stavudine and didanosine is decreased by co-administration with methadone. Similarly, when administering nelfinavir, methadone levels are reduced and so dosage adjustment is usually necessary. Some combinations such as ecstasy and ritonavir have proved fatal (Brettle 2001). It is important for clinicians to be aware of such possibilities.

In the antenatal period, it is good practice and can be reassuring for the mother to meet the paediatric team who will be involved in the follow-up care for her child. She may have particular questions about her baby's health as well as the practical issue of knowing where the clinic is. There may be particular issues that HIV positive pregnant women wish to discuss and specific antenatal classes have been established in some areas.

It is recommended that birth for an HIV positive woman at term should be by a pre-labour lower segment caesarean section (LSCS) as this has been shown to reduce significantly the risk of vertical transmission (European Mode of Delivery Collaboration 1999, International Perinatal HIV Group 1999).

She may have anxieties about the procedure, or about anaesthesia, which should be discussed and addressed in the antenatal period to allow her to make an informed choice. Zidovudine is given intravenously to the mother before and during the operation and the dosage is calculated on maternal weight. Other antiviral medication is given orally pre-operatively.

If the mother ruptures her membranes or goes into labour prematurely, the benefits of elective caesarean section are less clear and the risks of HIV transmission must be balanced with the risk of premature birth (Lyall et al 2001).

If a mother chooses vaginal birth, antiviral therapy should still be given, the membranes should be left intact for as long as possible, and fetal scalp electrodes and fetal blood sampling should be avoided. If there are signs of fetal distress, an emergency caesarean should be considered as the risk of vertical transmission is increased after emergency operative vaginal procedures (Lyall et al 2001).

The early postnatal period for any new mother is generally one of physical recovery from the birth combined with caring for and enjoying her newborn infant, and this should be no different for an HIV positive mother. Supporting her with recovery from a caesarean birth or from a vaginal birth and helping her care for her baby is an intrinsic part of midwifery care. There has been some evidence of poor wound healing with HIV infection and this should be monitored.

It can be distressing to women who are not breast feeding due to the risks of HIV infection if they lactate, and Cabergoline 1 milligram can be administered on the first postnatal day to assist suppression of lactation.

Women may also require assistance with bottle feeding, as they may never have done this before, even if they have had previous children. It is equally important that they are shown how to sterilise infant feeding equipment and prepare formula milk safely. Staff should ensure that women have access to supplies of formula milk, particularly after they leave hospital, and this may involve liaison with other HIV support services. For asylum seekers, who are not entitled to state assistance, this may be particularly difficult (Royal College of Midwives 2002).

The mother also needs to know how to administer antiviral drugs to the baby before she is discharged from the postnatal ward. Regimens will be explored in a later chapter but neonatal antiviral therapy is mainly dispensed in syrup form and needs to be drawn up, usually in a syringe (without a needle!) and given to the baby orally. This skill needs to be taught to the mother, and she must be given advice about the safe storage of the drug. Information about follow-up care for the woman and her baby, with appointment dates, times and venue should be given prior to discharge from the ward.

The mother will also need appropriate advice regarding contraception. This should include advice about safer sex and the prevention of transmission by the use of condoms as well as an additional method. Hormonal methods of contraception, particularly oral contraceptives, can have significant drug interactions with some antiviral drugs, resulting in either decreased contraceptive effectiveness or altered concentrations of the antiviral drug. For instance, nelfinavir, ritonavir, amprenavir and efavirenz may be associated with decreased effectiveness of oral contraceptives and increased breakthrough bleeding (Anderson 2000). It has been recommended that the intrauterine contraceptive device (IUCD) should be avoided in the context of HIV infection, as its use was linked to an increased risk for pelvic inflammatory disease, when women are at increased risk for acquiring other sexually transmitted diseases. Such infection could lead to an increased susceptibility to HIV transmission. However, more recent intrauterine systems (IUS such as Mirena) which contain the hormone progestogen, can be beneficial for this group of women and are not contraindicated.

Both intramuscular progesterone and progesterone implants are efficient contraceptives, though they may have interactions with antiretroviral therapy. Sterilisation may also be considered, though couples will still need to be advised about condom use to prevent transmission of sexually transmitted diseases (Bott 2000a).

Psychological health, counselling and support

As well as monitoring the physical health of the woman and her baby during pregnancy and childbirth, it is equally important to attend to her psychological and mental health needs. Initial responses to diagnosis may include shock, depression and anxiety about a number of issues. She may raise concerns about what will happen next in relation to her own health, her pregnancy and her child's health, or family relationships. These concerns may feel overwhelming to women, and it is important that organisations have support mechanisms in place. This may include a specialist midwife or obstetrician, health advisors, specialist nurses, counselling services, voluntary groups or community support groups. Some support groups are listed in Appendix 3.

Some individuals may also gain spiritual support from hospital chaplaincy services or their personal religious leaders.

Counselling involves understanding a person in their social and familial context and assisting them to develop coping strategies at a time when they are likely to be feeling vulnerable (Chippindale and French 2001).

Cultural norms will also influence the impact of an HIV diagnosis and pregnancy. For instance, the importance, in many cultures, of having a child should not be underestimated.

Support needs to be ongoing during pregnancy though some women will access it more frequently than others. The initial post-test counselling following a positive result is described elsewhere, but further follow-up is likely to revisit issues first raised at that appointment (Miller et al 1993).

The concerns for each HIV positive pregnant woman will be different, but common issues and questions raised may include:

● Their own health – will it deteriorate? If so, how quickly? How effective are the antiviral drugs and what are the possible side effects?
● Effect of HIV and also of stress on the pregnancy and the baby's health – 'Will my baby be all right?' There are likely to be particular anxieties for women who have an HIV positive child already, or who have had a previous child die of an HIV related illness.
● Effect on relationships – if they have told their partner about their infection, anxieties about his response and his test result if he has chosen to be tested; if they have not been able to tell him, anxieties about not telling him and living with a secret.
● Effect on family and other support network – 'How will they be if I tell them – will they support me and respect my confidentiality, ostracise me or tell all my community?'
● Anxieties about other family members – 'Are my other children infected? Should I have them tested? How will my parents react?'
● Decisions in pregnancy – not only 'Should I have a Caesarean, bottle feed and take antiviral therapy' but 'How will I explain it to people who do not know the real reason?'
● Effect on staff who care for them – 'how will they treat me? Who needs to know?'
● Welfare concerns, such as housing, finance or immigration issues.

This is not an exhaustive list and though the counsellor cannot 'solve all problems', counselling skills and techniques may help the woman to strengthen her own coping mechanisms (Chippindale and French 2001). Some women may have no family or friends that they feel they can turn to, and may have to rely solely on professional or voluntary support.

Even when women are aware of their HIV diagnosis before they become pregnant, they may still need to address issues or anxieties about HIV and pregnancy, or revisit issues about disclosure or their family support network.

If there are significant concerns about a woman's mental health, referral to appropriate psychiatric services should be offered.

It is important that women know how to access and contact counselling services, and that all staff maintain good liaison with other agencies in order to help address anxieties collaboratively.

Disclosure, confidentiality and documentation

In spite of advances in HIV medicine and greater public awareness about the infection, it remains a stigmatised illness, and one that can be difficult for women to talk about openly. It is recommended that the sexual partner of an infected individual is informed of the diagnosis in order to be offered counselling and screening for infection, treatment if appropriate and relevant sexual health promotion advice (NHPIS 2001). A separate appointment should be offered for the appropriate pre-test discussion and follow-up.

The process of partner notification can be patient/client-led or provider-led. The former approach is where the infected individual is encouraged to notify the partner and the latter where health care providers inform the partner on the basis of information provided by the infected person (SHASTD 2002).

This can be a very difficult decision for an individual to make, as he or she may be unsure of the partner's reaction. Whilst partners of some infected pregnant women have been supportive, domestic violence has been reported as well as rejection and lack of support during the pregnancy (Anderson 2000).

Issues regarding partner notification, and not telling a partner of the risk of infection, can arouse strong feelings as illustrated in a legal case where a man was found guilty of reckless behaviour for having unprotected sex with a woman, and not telling her when he knew he was HIV positive (Scott 2001).

If a woman feels unable to tell her partner, this decision must be respected, as health care workers have a duty of confidentiality regarding patient information unless there are exceptional circumstances (UKCC 1996, GMC 2000).

It is important not to pass judgement on the woman but to support her, and also to help her consider that her partner may question why she is taking antiviral therapy or not breast feeding if he is unaware of her infection. Any decisions about whether to tell other family members or friends rest with the woman.

Disclosure to staff involved in a woman's maternity care is based on a 'need to know' principle with the woman's consent. If no one in the maternity service is aware, appropriate antiviral therapy during the birth or timely referral of the baby to the paediatrician may be overlooked. Services have developed that involve a small team with whom the woman can develop a supportive and trusting relationship during pregnancy, birth and during the postnatal period. The involvement of the General Practitioner and the health visitor is recommended as they form an ongoing part of the health care team for the whole family. All health care workers involved have a professional duty of confidentiality regarding <u>all</u> health care information, including an individual's HIV status.

It is important that there are clear and informed channels of communication – both verbal and written. Verbal discussions should be held in private locations, not lift lobbies or other public areas. Written plans can be part of a birth plan that forms an additional part of the maternity records, as many mothers may be concerned with explicit documentation being included in their hand-held records, in case other family members read them. The mechanism for appropriate disclosure and documentation should be discussed and agreed with the woman.

It is clear that there are many overlapping issues that HIV positive pregnant women have to address. The aim is to balance the HIV care with that required for a healthy pregnancy, birth and postnatal period whilst allowing the woman to feel she has some control and support during these major life events.

Preconceptual care for couples already aware of their HIV status

While some women will learn for the first time of their HIV infection as a result of an antenatal screening test, others will be aware that they are HIV positive prior to pregnancy. The decision to consider embarking upon a pregnancy has been partly attributed to the improved prognosis for infected adults and the interventions available to reduce vertical transmission. It is important that health care workers can give appropriate preconceptual advice to couples in this position, whether or not they choose ultimately to have a child. Such couples may either be:

● An HIV positive man and an HIV negative woman
● An HIV negative man and an HIV positive woman

Such couples may be described in the literature as discordant couples.

Additionally there may be couples where both the man and the woman are HIV positive.

Standard preconceptual advice should be provided for all couples, and this should include recommendations on smoking cessation, appropriate diet and the use of folic acid as well as specific advice in relation to HIV infection. For the partner who is HIV positive it is important to establish what the viral load and CD4 count is and what antiviral therapy he or she is taking, as the drug regime may need alteration. There is some evidence that HIV may have an adverse effect on fertility in both symptomatic and asymptomatic women (Anderson 2000) and appropriate investigations may need to be arranged.

As with any couple planning a family, there are no guarantees of a pregnancy and such a possibility should also be discussed. The Human Fertilisation and Embryology Authority (HFEA) provides guidance regarding counselling before embarking on assisted conception programmes, that include consideration of the welfare of the child, and these apply in the context of HIV infection as well (HFEA 2001).

For discordant couples there is the risk of sexual transmission of HIV. This risk may be reduced for HIV negative women by limiting exposure to seminal fluid to the most fertile period, and by the use of a technique known as 'sperm washing'. In this process, spermatozoa are removed from the surrounding HIV infected seminal fluid by a 'swim up' technique. The 'washed' sperm is then inseminated into the negative woman. There have been no seroconversions so far in women receiving this treatment (Semprini et al 1992, Lyall et al 2001). However, they may still have anxieties about seroconversion during the pregnancy. Where the woman is HIV positive and the man HIV negative, artificial insemination can be performed by the couple at the time of ovulation using quills, syringes, gallipots or 'turkey basters'.

The advice when both partners are positive is to practice unprotected intercourse during the fertile period.

Opinions about whether infertile couples with HIV should be treated have altered with the advent of antiviral therapy and lower vertical transmission rates (Gilling-Smith et al 2001). Following conception, the same levels of support and advice as for any other couple affected by HIV will be required.

Summary

Care for an HIV positive woman and her family, whether before or after conception, is diverse and multifaceted. Areas it needs to address include:

- Her physical care, both generally and in relation to her HIV infection.
- Her pregnancy care from conception through the pregnancy and birth to the postnatal period.
- Her emotional and psychological wellbeing, including her response to diagnosis, and support to develop coping strategies for dealing with the implications of pregnancy and infection.
- The social and cultural aspects of her life, and how HIV and pregnancy may impact on them.
- The clear and informed channels of communication between the woman and those directly involved in her care.

Chapter 8

Care of the infant

In addition to the care that all newborn infants require, there are specific points that are particularly relevant to the baby of an HIV positive mother. These include:

- diagnostic testing
- feeding the baby
- antiviral therapy for the infant
- prophylactic therapy for the infant against Pneumocystis carinii pneumonia (PCP)
- psychosocial support for the family
- paediatric follow-up care
- care for the HIV positive child.

Diagnostic testing for the infant

The first question parents ask after the birth of a child may be: 'Is he/she all right?' When the mother is HIV positive, the significance of this question is increased, as testing will need to occur before it can be fully answered.

Infants are described as of 'indeterminate HIV status' until definitive results are known.

Initial, baseline blood tests should be taken from the baby as soon as possible after birth, and prior to neonatal antiviral therapy being administered. Investigations required include HIV DNA polymerase chain reaction (PCR), which is the 'gold standard' test for HIV infection in infancy. Whilst HIV DNA is not genetically amplified from all infected infants at birth, by three months of age more than 95% of non-breast fed HIV infected infants will be PCR positive (Lyall et al 2001). HIV RNA PCR and HIV culture may also be used in certain circumstances. It is important to have close liaison with the appropriate laboratories so that specimens are acted upon promptly. Current practice in a number of units is to test the infant at:

- birth (24-48 hours)
- one month
- three months.

If all HIV PCR testing is negative at these stages, the parents are informed that the child is not infected. Otherwise, antibody testing is carried out at 18 months.

HIV antibody testing of an infant is not a diagnostic test for him or her as all babies born to infected women will have passively acquired IgG antibodies to HIV. The median length of time for the infant to lose this antibody is 10 months but it may be as long as 18 months. However, it is recommended that antibody testing be performed at the 18 months period to ensure that sero-reversion has occurred.

Further annual follow-up is recommended for HIV negative children who have been exposed to maternal antiviral therapy in utero to assess for any possible long-term side effects.

Other tests recommended in the first 24-48 hours are full blood count and white blood cell differential, a urine sample to exclude cytomegalovirus infection, hepatitis B and C serology if relevant. A liver function test may also be suggested (Gibb 1998a).

Many parents find blood testing on a baby distressing and staff should be sensitive to this and provide clear explanations as part of the consent procedure.

Feeding the baby

In the United Kingdom formula feeding is recommended for infants born to HIV positive mothers to reduce the risk of vertical transmission of HIV. Although it can be a difficult decision to make, most mothers agree to it.

It is important that they receive support with formula feeding, both in the practical skills involved, including sterilisation of feeding equipment and preparing formula feeds, as well as access to regular supplies of formula milk, particularly after discharge from the postnatal ward. If the mother is entitled to certain state welfare benefits, such as income support, she is likely to be able to access milk tokens that can be exchanged for milk powder. However, if she is not entitled to state support, and has little or no income, she may be unable to afford formula milk. This has been particularly highlighted in the case of HIV positive asylum seekers (Royal College of Midwives 2002) who are not eligible for income support. Some health and local authorities and voluntary groups have established feeding schemes to ensure that all HIV positive mothers have regular access to milk supplies.

A highly publicised case in the late 1990s of an HIV positive mother who chose to breast feed and declined testing for her baby was brought to court by a Social Services department under the remit of child protection legislation. Following a court ruling that the child should be tested for HIV, the parents and their daughter fled the country (Brahams 1999). They returned following the death of the mother, and the diagnosis of infection in the daughter (Boseley 2002).

This case raised a number of issues about child protection and HIV in relation to testing the infant, breast feeding and declining treatment.

It is essential that open and ongoing communication continues between parents and all services involved in such a difficult and emotive aspect of care, and recommendations for good practice have been drawn up (Pan London Local Authority Children and Families HIV Consultation Forum 2000).

Antiviral therapy for the infant

The recommended antiviral regimen for an infant born to an HIV positive mother will depend on various factors including what therapy she has been taking in pregnancy, and what her viral load and CD4 count levels are prior to delivery. Although, in the 076 study, zidovudine was administered to the baby four times a day for six weeks, shorter courses have been shown to be effective (Lallemant et al 2000). In United Kingdom centres, neonates are currently treated for 4-6 weeks, commonly with monotherapy of zidovudine.

It is not known whether combination therapy for the infant has any additional benefit over single drug treatment, in situations where the infant's infection status is not yet known. However, combination therapy for the infant should be considered if a mother delivers prematurely prior to starting antiretroviral therapy, is diagnosed late in pregnancy or soon after delivery before details of her viral load and other markers are available, or if she has declined treatment during pregnancy (Lyall et al 2001).

Once a decision has been agreed as to which antiviral drugs are suitable for the infant, they should be prescribed (based on infant weight) and then administered appropriately. As soon as the mother feels physically able after the birth, she should be taught how to measure and administer the correct dose, and this is best carried out before a feed.

It is also important that the mother is aware of the possibility of short-term or long-term side effects, what to look out for, and who to contact. Rashes, diarrhoea and vomiting or signs of anaemia can all be significant.

Prophylactic therapy against Pneumocystis carinii pneumonia (PCP)

PCP occurs most frequently in infants under six months of age who are immune suppressed, and it has a high mortality rate. It is recommended that PCP prophylaxis commences as soon as neonatal zidovudine is stopped (4-6 weeks) and continues either until infection status is clearly negative or for the first year of life in infected children (Gibb 1998a). Co-trimoxazole is the drug of choice.

More recently, with the reduction in vertical transmission rates to <1% it is felt that the need for PCP prophylaxis has declined, and many European countries no longer prescribe it (Lyall et al 2001).

Psychosocial support for the family

Waiting for an infant's diagnosis can be a stressful time as, even though the rate of vertical transmission is low when interventions are taken up, there is still uncertainty regarding the child's result in the first few months of life. Such uncertainty may affect or delay mother-infant attachment. Anxiety regarding the infant's health may also be increased if the mother has had a previous child who was infected. If the child is HIV negative, parents may still have concerns about who would look after their child if they became ill, and professionals should be sensitive to such anxieties and refer to appropriate agencies where necessary. If the child or the mother requires hospital admission, services such as rooming-in facilities on paediatric wards, or units such as the Mildmay family unit in London, where children can stay with their parents, can help reduce to reduce separation anxiety.

Paediatric follow-up care

The issues of diagnostic testing, antiviral therapy and prophylactic treatment against opportunistic infections are all key elements of paediatric follow-up care for the infant of an HIV positive mother. They should all be addressed alongside standard monitoring of infant growth and development that may occur in a hospital or community clinic. Parents are encouraged to allow the General Practitioner and health visitor to be informed of the diagnosis so that they can base health assessments on appropriate knowledge, and provide additional, appropriate support if parents are awaiting test results or have other anxieties relating to their child's health.

Infants born to HIV infected mothers should partake in the national routine immunisation schedule, except that BCG should not be given until the infant is confirmed uninfected. There has been concern that giving live oral polio vaccine to HIV infected infants could prove a risk to them and their carers, and that 'killed' polio vaccine should be given by injection instead. However, the risk of oral polio vaccine has not been shown to be significant, and most infants will usually have had two negative PCR test results by eight weeks, so this precaution is unnecessary (Lyall et al 2001).

Care for the HIV positive child

This is only a brief overview of paediatric HIV. For more detail the reader is referred to specific paediatric texts (Pizzo and Wilfert 1998).

It is likely to be rare (<2%) that an infant is HIV positive if the mother has received treatment recommended during pregnancy, at birth and in the postnatal period. A positive result, in these circumstances, is likely to be a shock to the parents and appropriate specialist support will be required from paediatric and other services.

In addition, diagnosis of paediatric HIV infection may occur when a child presents with symptoms to paediatric services.

Such symptoms include:

- PCP in infancy leading to severe respiratory failure (though this is less common with earlier diagnosis and improvements in paediatric intensive care).
- Widespread lymphadenopathy, recurrent bacterial infections, diarrhoea and failure to thrive which pre-school children most commonly present with. Bilateral persistent parotid enlargement is also a useful sign of HIV infection.
- Opportunistic infections or organ disease such as isolated cardiomyopathy or chronic renal failure.
(Sharland 2001).

As part of the differential diagnosis of children presenting with such symptoms, HIV testing should be discussed and offered. Consent is always required before a child can have an HIV test, and as with adults such consent should be informed. Where a child has reached the age of 16 years he or she is deemed to be capable of giving or refusing consent to their own medical treatment, but this may also apply to younger children if they are of sufficient age, maturity and understanding (previously described as 'Gillick competent'). Where children are considered too young or otherwise unable to understand, consent must be gained from the parent or guardian (Department of Health 2001d).

Where testing is agreed to, clear explanations and reassurance should be given, and it is good practice to use local anaesthetic creams prior to phlebotomy in children.

When a woman is diagnosed in pregnancy, the issue of testing any other children should be raised as part of the ongoing post-test counselling with the appropriate involvement of paediatric services.

Management of HIV infection in children follows similar principles to management in adults in terms of monitoring the infection, the use of antiviral therapy and psychosocial and counselling support (Pizzo and Wilfert 1998).

However, there are differences between children and adults with HIV disease and guidelines have been produced for the use of antiretroviral therapy in paediatric infection (Sharland et al 2001a). These date rapidly and clinicians are advised to talk to specialists in this area and keep updated from relevant websites such as the Paediatric European Network for Treatment of AIDS (PENTA) www.ctu.mrc.ac.uk/penta.

Significant progress has been made in treating HIV infection in children and mortality rates are declining.

As well as challenges about what to prescribe and how to ensure adherence, issues about when and how to tell a child his or her diagnosis, or that of their parent(s), as well as the differing needs of children of different ages are complex areas of paediatric HIV care. For example, as children with HIV survive into adolescence, specific support services have been developed such as Teen Spirit – a London-based self-help group for young people aged 13 years and over who know their own HIV status or that of their family (www.bodyandsoul.demon.co.uk).

Whatever the age of the child, and whether they are infected with or affected by HIV, it is important to be aware of and sensitive to their particular needs and those of their parents and families.

Summary

- HIV DNA PCR testing is the gold standard test for HIV infection in infancy.
- Current practice is to test the infant at birth, one month and three months of age. If all HIV DNA PCR results are negative at these stages the infant is not infected. In addition, HIV negative children who have been exposed to maternal antiretroviral therapy before and during birth should be followed up annually for any long-term side effects.
- HIV antibody testing in an infant is not a diagnostic test, due to passive transfer of maternal antibodies across the placenta. HIV antibody testing should be performed on HIV PCR negative children at 18 months of age to ensure sero-reversion.
- Formula feeding is recommended for infants born to HIV positive mothers to reduce the risk of vertical transmission. This decision can be difficult to make, and mothers should receive appropriate support.
- Antiviral therapy is recommended for infants, and the choice of drug is based on a number of factors. As soon as practical parents should be taught how to administer the drug(s) safely to their child.
- Antibiotic prophylaxis against Pneumocystis carinii pneumonia (PCP) is recommended, either until infection status is confirmed as negative, or for the first year of life in infected children.
- There can be considerable anxiety waiting for a child's diagnosis, and this may delay or otherwise affect mother-infant attachment.

Health care workers and others involved should be sensitive to such anxieties.

● Standard child health and development assessments, including participation in appropriate immunisation programmes, are part of follow-up care for infants. Parents are encouraged to allow the General Practitioner, health visitor or other relevant members of the family's health care team to be informed of the diagnosis.

● HIV testing in all children, whatever their age, requires informed consent either from the parent or guardian, or from the child where possible. If a mother is recently diagnosed in pregnancy, information regarding testing of other children should be included as part of post-test counselling.

● Management of an HIV infected child follows similar principles to that of adults. However there are important differences and referral to the latest paediatric guidelines on antiretroviral therapy and to specialist paediatric services is essential.

Chapter 9

Health care workers and HIV infection

All health care workers, including those in the maternity services, need to understand the implications of HIV infection in order to provide appropriate information and care to women, and for their own professional practice. This chapter will describe:

- The risk of HIV infection for the health care worker through occupational exposure, and measures to reduce such risks
- Issues and advice for HIV infected health care workers
- The importance of training about HIV infection for all health care workers.

Occupational risks of HIV infection for health care workers

HIV is a fragile organism outside of the body, easily inactivated by normal domestic hygiene measures. Accidental inoculation with HIV positive blood, known as a percutaneous injury, is estimated to have a 0.3% risk of infection compared to a risk of 30% with the Hepatitis B virus. Mucocutaneous injuries, or exposure of the mucous membranes and/or conjunctivae are estimated to have a lower risk of HIV transmission of 0.03%.

Up to 1999, there had been 102 cases worldwide of health care workers in whom seroconversion was documented after occupational exposure to HIV (PHLS 1999).

Recommendations have been made to try and reduce the risk of occupational exposure to body fluids and blood borne infections (see box 9.1).

Box 9.1

● Wash hands before and after contact with each patient, and before and after removing gloves.

● Change gloves between patients.

● Cover existing wounds, skin lesions and all breaks in exposed skin with waterproof dressings. Wear gloves if hands are extensively affected.

● Wear gloves where contact with blood can be anticipated.

● Avoid 'sharps' usage where possible, and where 'sharps' usage is essential, exercise particular care in handling and disposal.

● Avoid wearing open footwear in situations where blood may be spilt, or where sharp instruments or needles are handled.

● Clear up spillage of blood promptly and disinfect surfaces.

● Wear gloves when cleaning equipment prior to sterilisation or disinfection, when handling chemical disinfectants, and when cleaning up spillages.

● Follow safe procedures for disposal of contaminated waste according to appropriate Health and Safety guidance.

(Department of Health 1998)

Particular care needs to be taken when using sharp instruments, and needles should <u>never</u> be resheathed but discarded immediately after use. Safer phlebotomy procedures have been adopted whereby sample bottles can be filled directly whilst the needle remains in the vein. When all samples have been taken, the needle and holder are removed without any disconnection being required, and disposed of in an approved sharps box. Such containers, which should be used for the disposal of all 'sharps', should not be overfilled and when they are two-thirds full should be replaced.

In addition, the use of eyewear to protect the mucous membrane of the eyes is recommended in situations where splashing of body fluids may be anticipated. Some midwives have stated that the wearing of barrier precautions, especially eye protection, could create a barrier in the relationship with the woman during labour and delivery (Grellier et al 1996). However, this assumption needs further examination, and the views of women should be sought.

What appears fundamental, however, is that high standards of infection control must be applied universally, not selectively, in the care for all women, in order to avoid discriminatory practice whilst ensuring the protection of staff. There is evidence that such precautions have not been universally adopted (Grellier et al 1996).

Implementation of such precautions will be facilitated by:

- Clear practice guidelines for all team members that are widely disseminated and regularly updated.
- A well-planned work environment including the use of appropriate equipment to minimise the risk of occupational injury.
- Role models of good infection control practice within the clinical area.
- Effective and regular staff training and education programmes regarding Universal Infection Control Precautions.
- Monitoring and audit of practice, and investigation when injuries occur to see if any trends emerge. (Bott 1999)

Accidental occupational exposure – what to do

There are recommended procedures to be adopted if a health care worker is accidentally exposed to blood or body fluids during clinical practice, usually as a result of a needlestick or splash injury, and every employer should draw up a policy on the management of exposures (Department of Health 1998). Immediate action includes:

- Washing the wound or non-intact skin liberally with soap and water without scrubbing.
- Irrigating exposed mucous membranes, including conjunctivae, copiously with water, before and after removing contact lenses if present.
- Encouraging free bleeding, if there has been a puncture wound, by gentle squeezing (but not sucking) of the wound.

Following this, the health care worker should report the exposure promptly and seek further advice on management and treatment from a designated team. This team will usually include colleagues from the occupational health department, virology or other laboratory services.

An assessment of risk of blood borne virus transmission will be carried out. Such assessments include:

● Information about the source patient including risk factors for blood borne viral infections and any appropriate test results where known. The source patient should be asked to consent to testing for infections including HIV, Hepatitis B and C. If they are approached in a sensitive manner and receive full pre-test discussion, it is understood that consent to testing is rarely withheld (Department of Health 1998). Such discussion should be carried out by a person other than the individual who has received the injury, to avoid undue anxiety or pressure accompanying the request for testing.

● If the source patient is known to be infected with HIV, then information regarding their current HIV viral load and past and current antiviral therapy will also be required.

● Information about the injury and an assessment of the level of exposure will need to be made. This includes information regarding the type of needlestick injury or the level of mucocutaneous exposure.

Although the risk of acquiring HIV infection through occupational exposure is low (0.03-0.3%), when such situations occur they are frequently very stressful for the member of staff involved. Information, counselling and psychological support should be available for any employee who reports such an exposure, and during the follow-up period.

Post-exposure prophylaxis for health care workers

If a health care worker has an occupational exposure to HIV, post-exposure prophylaxis (PEP) of antiviral therapy is available. Guidelines have been developed by the Expert Advisory Group on AIDS (EAGA) regarding the use of antiviral therapy in such situations (Department of Health 2000c).

These guidelines include advice on assessment of risk, when PEP should be recommended, the choice of antiviral drugs, how to ensure that all health care workers have immediate 24-hour access to advice, drugs and appropriate support, and the setting up of local policies and protocols.

At present, the recommended drugs for PEP are zidovudine, lamivudine and indinavir or nelfinavir. They should be taken for four weeks. However, allowances must be made for viral resistance in the source patient, drug interactions or pregnancy in the affected health care worker, so that the regimen may be modified. Such information regarding antiviral therapy and its use will be constantly changing, and expert advice should be sought when injuries occur. It is essential that all staff are aware of the process, and of how to access such advice whenever it is required.

HIV positive health care workers

If a health care worker is infected with HIV, by whatever route of transmission, they are entitled to expect that their confidentiality will be respected and protected. They also have an ethical, legal and professional duty to protect the health and safety of the people in their care. Concerns have been raised that an infected health care worker could transmit HIV infection to a patient through clinical practice, and that even though the risk is small, patients should be informed of it (Blatchford et al 2000).

No cases of transmission of HIV infection from health care worker to patient through clinical practice have ever been detected in the United Kingdom, despite 22 extensive 'look back' exercises (Department of Health 2001c). There have been only two reported cases worldwide: a dentist in Florida, where HIV was transmitted to six patients, though the exact route of transmission has never been established, and an infected orthopaedic surgeon in France who transmitted HIV to a patient.

'Look back' exercises involve identifying and notifying patients who had had an exposure-prone procedure performed on them by a health care worker who was subsequently diagnosed with HIV infection. Testing was offered to these patients, but no cases of occupational transmission were confirmed.

In the light of these findings, the guidance on patient notification has been altered, and will be assessed on a case-by-case basis. This is in line with policy in the rest of the world (Department of Health 2001c).

If a health care worker believes that they may have been exposed to infection with HIV, they must seek professional advice on whether they should be tested for HIV infection. If diagnosed positive, they should inform the occupational health department. The Midwives Rules and Code of Practice (Rule 39) requires midwives to be medically examined if necessary to prevent the spread of infection (UKCC 1998a).

Support and confidentiality is as essential for the HIV infected health care worker as it is for any other individual with an HIV diagnosis, and appropriate guidance should be referred to (UK Health Departments 1999, Royal College of Midwives 1998). HIV positive midwives are advised not to perform certain exposure-prone procedures such as suturing of an episiotomy, and such restrictions may require employers to arrange suitable alternative work or retraining options for infected staff. Such discussions will need to be handled sensitively.

Staff training

Information for health care workers about HIV infection and how it could affect their practice should be included in staff training programmes for students and qualified staff. Knowledge and attitudes may vary, and affects how confident health care workers feel in their approach to this infection (Bruce et al 2001, Duffy and Moore 2000, Scoular et al 2000, Grellier et al 1996).

Regular update sessions are important in this changing field, and can be provided by formal or informal teaching sessions, appropriate journal reviews and Internet sites.

Summary

In conclusion, it is important that health care workers have an understanding of HIV for their own professional practice.

- A health care worker who receives a percutaneous (contaminated sharp instrument) injury with HIV positive blood is estimated to have a 0.3% risk of acquiring infection. The risk with a mucocutaneous injury (exposure of the mucous membranes) is estimated to be lower at 0.03% risk.
- To reduce the risk of occupational exposure to body fluids and blood borne infections, universal infection control precautions (UICP) should always be applied.

- Implementation of IUCP requires clear and widely disseminated practice guidelines, the use of appropriate equipment, regular staff training and monitoring, and audit of practice and investigation when injuries occur.
- If there is an exposure, first aid measures include washing the wound liberally with soap and water, or irrigating mucous membranes with water. If there has been a puncture wound free bleeding should be encouraged by squeezing. The incident should be reported promptly and appropriate advice sought.
- Further follow-up of the source patient and the nature of the injury will form part of the assessment of the exposure and risk of transmission.
- If a health care worker has an occupational exposure to HIV, post-exposure prophylaxis (PEP) of antiviral therapy is available. Prompt expert advice should be sought.
- All health care workers have an ethical, legal and professional duty to protect the health and safety of the people in their care.
- No cases of transmission from an HIV positive health care worker to a patient through clinical practice have ever been detected in the United Kingdom.
- Guidance on patient notification is on a case-by-case basis.
- If a midwife is diagnosed HIV positive, he or she should seek occupational health advice and has a requirement to be medically examined.
- HIV positive health care workers are advised not to perform exposure-prone procedures. Such restrictions may require employers to arrange suitable alternative work or retraining options for infected staff.
- Support and confidentiality is as essential for the HIV infected health care worker as it is for any other individual with an HIV diagnosis.
- Regular training is important for all staff and can be from a variety of sources.

Chapter 10

Personal perspectives

All of us who are health care professionals need to listen to what our patients, in this instance the women in our care, tell us. They are the experts on their experience of HIV and of how they are feeling, not us. This book would not be complete without their contribution, and the following accounts were written by women with whom I have worked, and from whom I have learned so much.

All of the names have been changed to protect the identity of the women concerned; no other alterations have been made.

Julie's story

My name is Julie.

A few years ago I had thrush in my mouth. It wasn't painful but it bothered me so I went to my GP who gave me something for it. It wasn't getting better so after going back to my GP several times he referred me to a dermatologist. One of the questions she asked me was whether I had ever had a test for HIV as it could be related. I said: 'No – I don't have that, so no, I don't want to have the test.' She suggested it would be a good thing to know if I did have it but encouraged me to go home and think about it.

When I was at home I was quite down. I thought: No – I don't have this, and that I would die if I did, so I didn't want to test. The doctor contacted me at home to ask if I had given it any more thought. Eventually, after a few more phone calls, I encouraged myself to go and see a health advisor to discuss it. I decided to have the test.

I was to return for the result in a week but when I got home I became down again and thought: What would I do if the result was positive? I'm not ill, so I'm not positive, so I won't go for the result.

I did go back for the result – it was positive. I kept quiet for several minutes and my heart was pounding. Then I cried and cried. I felt it was a death certificate. I was shocked: Maybe it's a mistake. I will do a repeat test and then see.

I remember I asked the health advisor: What about children – can I still have them? When she said I could still have them, and that by doing various things there were chances that a baby could be negative, I was really happy.

After my result I didn't want to tell anyone I felt ashamed – maybe they would think I was going to die tomorrow. I was even worried that my two friends who used the same GP as me would know.

I wanted to start treatment straight away but had to wait for the results of my CD4 counts and viral load test which took about 3 weeks. While I was waiting I read loads of leaflets about the drugs, the side effects, all sorts of things.

I had mixed feelings: I wanted treatment but I was surprised that it would be 'medication for life' – I knew I wasn't good at remembering to take medication every day.

I still remember my first results: CD4 count of 62 (which is low) and a viral load of 124,000 (which is high).

I started taking medication (Combivir and Nevirapine) which the doctor said was good for young women who were thinking of having children. I had some side effects of vomiting, headaches, rashes, some fever and a bitter taste in my mouth, which I had been told about, but these settled down after about two weeks.

I went back to the clinic every month to see how I was doing. After 3 months my viral load was coming down a bit and after 6 months it was undetectable.

Oh, and my mouth had cleared up completely. I thought: Maybe I will live till next month.

It was still in my mind that I wanted a child. I had a miscarriage during my first year of treatment but although I was very disappointed and sad, by this time I had educated myself about HIV and pregnancy and knew that it wasn't necessarily connected to my illness.

However, about 6 months later I became pregnant again and I was happy to be pregnant although I wasn't sure it was the right time as I thought my CD4 count should have been at least 500 and it was only 280!

Though I was excited to be pregnant, being positive put me down. What would I do if the baby was positive?

I knew about the interventions and agreed to all of them – the planned caesarean, the medication which I was already on and not breast feeding.

Not breast feeding was hard, especially when you hear messages like children who are breast fed are brighter. I sometimes felt guilty being positive and worried that the medication might affect the baby. I sometimes got a bit confused like that AZT is often used for HIV positive pregnant women but I was on Combivir and Nevirapine – though in fact Combivir is a mixture of AZT and 3TC.

I had my baby, a boy, and he is lovely. He has now had three clear results so I'm very happy. I feel so guilty when he has blood taken as he cries and cries and they have to squeeze to get the blood out. I was worried that he might be ill in the first three months. When the doctor told me he is negative, I was happy but worried – what is going to happen next time?

I have told my partner and my sister who have both been very understanding and helpful with me and with my son. I think about telling my mum but as my dad died not long ago I don't think now is the right time.

When I think about testing I think that all women should have the test as you really don't know. You think it happens to others, not me.

For now, I'm taking each day as it comes. At the moment I'm doing very well and so is my son. I would like more children, but not just yet. I hope they will find medication for a cure, as to take medication every day is hard and reminds me that I'm positive.

Mandy's story

In February 1997 while lying in my hospital bed, not getting any better after having twins, I was asked if they could test me for HIV. Sure, I said, not thinking for one minute of what the result would be, after all I never did drugs or slept around. All the things any sensible person should do, I did. Well, when Jane came back a few days later with the results, I knew straight away it was positive; you see, Jane has that kind of face – if she ever played poker she would probably end up homeless.

The worse thing was that while I was pregnant they asked if I wanted to be tested, I said yes and for some unknown reason they never did it. Believe me, if they had I would certainly have terminated my pregnancy without a second thought.

Being in a room on my own never helped, I felt isolated and so alone at times. I just wanted to turn the clocks back and start all over again. Every now and again someone would go past and open the little glass flaps to look in, start whispering amongst themselves, making you feel dirty and cheap, it made me feel as if I was in a sideshow. You know: 'That's the one who tested positive' -made me feel like I was some kind of freak. Sure there were some really great nurses in there and they treated me no different than any other patient but there was also some who would be too afraid to even come in the room.

The next 18 months were a living nightmare, waiting to see if my babies were positive or not. If they got a cold or anything then I'd panic, luckily for me they came back negative. Now I could finally start making plans for them to go to school and arrange for someone to take care of them if I wasn't around for it. I've still made certain provisions for them just in case. At the moment my health is good and the medication seems to be working, for how long I don't know. So I live from day to day and thank God that I am well enough to be able to take care of them. Hopefully I'll be around for a long time yet, but there are no guarantees with this disease even though they are coming up with new drugs every so often.

Who knows, maybe someday they will even find a cure for it, maybe not in my lifetime, but in the next generation's lifetime. Nearly five years on and I still find it hard to come to terms with, thinking 'Why me?' I also at times regret agreeing to be tested, and then I think: 'Well, what if I never got tested. Would I still be here? My kids would have no mother to look out for them, to cuddle them when they fall over and hurt themselves, or to kiss them goodnight and tell them how much I love them.'

I am lucky in some ways because I have the support of the members of my family who know I am positive. They have not changed their opinion of me and love me for who I am and not what I have. Not everyone has that luxury and some are shunned by the people they thought they could rely on in times of need and trouble. If I never had my family I really don't know if I would be here today, as this is not something you can deal with on your own. I was lucky I had my family and even my GP for support. Even the doctors and nurses at the clinic I attend are absolutely brilliant, and treat you with respect and not like something that you have just scraped off the bottom of your shoe. I even keep in contact with the 'grim reaper'. That was the nickname I came up with for dear old Jane, the bearer of my bad news that knocked me for six.

When I look at my angels sleeping I just pray that I am around to see them achieve their goals in life, whatever they may be. So long as they are happy then I'm happy; what more can I ask for. I have two beautiful children who are healthy and are about to start school and that is something I never dreamt of seeing.

Maybe it's God's will that I was never tested when I was pregnant, who knows what he has in store for us in this life or even in the next life. I'm just grateful to still be here, alive and in fairly good health.

Liz's story

Mark had a urine infection and was referred to hospital where we were both given treatment and offered to take the HIV test. Five months after the test Mark went for his results, which he said were negative. I went for mine which I was told was positive. I could not believe my ears – so much so that I had to ask the Health Advisor to repeat himself. I sat there sobbing, numb, confused, angry and hurting all at the same time. The Health Advisor was going on about treatment and support but I wasn't interested. My mind was spinning and I began to feel dizzy. I was 14 weeks pregnant, how could I not feel dizzy!

I was referred to a specialist clinic the same day and told I would be managed by a midwife who is experienced in HIV and pregnancy. An appointment to see the midwife and the doctor who was going to look after me was made.

On my way home, I was wondering whether to tell Mark the devastating news or to keep it to myself. I asked myself so many questions: 'Am I dying?' 'What will happen to Julie (my 6 year old daughter from a previous marriage) when I die' (considering that I had no contact with her dad) and 'How will my family, especially my mum, cope when I'm dead, being the bread winner.' I wondered how I'll look like when I have full blown AIDS. Will I look like those people I've seen on TV? I thought of committing suicide but the one thing that would stop me was Julie. I wouldn't want my Julie to suffer so I had to be strong for myself and her.

Breaking the news to Mark was one of the most difficult things I'd ever done. All Mark said was 'I don't believe it'. We both cried most of the night as it was really a shock. Mark suggested we take another test at a different hospital. We did, and again he was negative and I was positive. I was devastated. Mark tried to support me as much as he could. We decided we had to attend the specialist clinic as advised.

Attending the clinic was not as bad as I'd thought. The staff were all lovely and very supportive which was all I needed. Deciding to have a C section, taking AZT and not breast feeding was not difficult for me. The doctors told me other women had had HIV negative babies by taking treatment, C section and not breast feeding and so I started taking AZT at 24 weeks. I had had a positive Heaf test so I was also taking anti-TB drugs. I'd take $4^1/_2$ tablets per day: 2 medium-sized capsules before food early in the morning plus half a tablet to stop side effects, 1 capsule (AZT) at 10 am and the last AZT at 10pm. The anti-TB medicine took 12 weeks and I took AZT for 14 weeks. For all those weeks I was never sick, simply because I told myself I didn't have to be.

My worries from the day I knew I was positive were who would look after my children if I die. I was told that, with treatment, I could live for many years but still at the back of my mind I knew my life span had been shortened by the virus. I was worried about Mark as well. He'd avoid talking about it and I didn't know why. I wondered what was going on in his mind – did he think I was a 'loose' person, was he going to leave me for someone HIV negative?

All Mark said was 'Don't worry – everything will be all right.'

I was lucky to have brilliant midwives. My favourite midwife made me feel a lot better and confident. I looked forward to my appointments, hoping to be attended to by her. At the time I was almost having a nervous breakdown – she saved me. She automatically took my Mum's place as I'd open up to her my innermost feelings. She let me cry when I needed to, and the best thing was she seemed not to mind my being HIV positive.

Seven months have gone now since I was diagnosed. I feel stronger and think positively. I have to be there for my family as they need me as much as I need them. Little Adrian was born weighing 3kg and is healthy. He was tested at birth and was negative. He still has to take more tests which I hope and pray will be negative too. Julie also took the test, as the doctors advised, and I was relieved because she is negative. I still cry a lot at times though I try to be as happy as I can. It's always there, at the back of my mind, but it does not stop me smiling and thanking God each morning I wake up!

References

Adler M W 2001 ABC of AIDS, 5th edn. BMJ Books, London

Aldeen T, Wells C, Hay P et al 1999 Lipodystrophy associated with nevirapine containing antiretroviral therapies. AIDS 13 (7): 865-866

Alexander N J 1996 Sexual spread of HIV infection. European Society of Human Reproduction and Embryology 11 (Supplement): 111-120

Anderson J 2000 Guide to the care of women with HIV infection: HIV and reproduction. U.S. Dept of Health and Human Services, Rockville, MD

Andreasson P A, Dias F, Naucler A et al 1993 A prospective study of vertical transmission of HIV 2 in Bissau, Guinea-Bissau. AIDS 7: 989-993

Ashurst P, Hall Z 1989 Understanding women in distress. Tavistock/Routledge, London/New York

Association of British Insurers 1994 ABI statement of practice: underwriting life insurance for HIV/AIDS. ABI, London

Barre-Sinoussi F, Cherman J C, Rey F et al 1983 Isolation of a T-lymphotrophic retrovirus from a patient at risk for acquired immune deficiency syndrome (AIDS). Science 220 (4599): 868-871

Bastow V 2000 Identifying and treating PCP. Nursing Times Plus 96 (37): 19-20

Baxter J, Bennett R 2000 What do pregnant women think about antenatal HIV testing? RCM Midwives Journal 3 (10): 308-311

Bessinger R, Clark R, Kissinger P et al 1998 Pregnancy is not associated with the progression of HIV disease in women attending an HIV outpatient programme. American Journal of Epidemiology 147: 434-440

Beverley P, Helbert M 2001 Immunology of AIDS. In: Adler M W (ed) ABC of AIDS 5th edn. BMJ Books, London

Biggar R J, Miotto P G, Taha T E et al 1996 Perinatal intervention trial in Africa: effect of a birth canal cleansing intervention to prevent HIV transmission. Lancet 347: 1647-1650

Blanche S, Tardieu M, Rustin P et al 1999 Persistent mitochondrial dysfunction and perinatal exposure to antiretroviral nucleoside analogues. Lancet 354: 1084-1089

Blatchford O, O'Brien S J, Blatchford M et al 2000 Infectious health care workers: should patients be told? Journal of Medical Ethics 26: 27-33

Boseley S 2002 HIV girl to be brought back to UK. The Guardian 4 May

Bott J 1999 HIV risk reduction and the use of universal precautions. British Journal of Midwifery 7 (11): 671-675

Bott J 2000 HIV screening during pregnancy: gender issues. British Journal of Midwifery 8 (3): 174-177

Bott J 2000a HIV and women: health and childbearing issues. British Journal of Midwifery 8 (1): 15-19

Boyd F, Simpson W M, Hart G J et al 1999b What do pregnant women think about the HIV test? AIDS Care 11 (1): 21-29

Boyd F, Simpson W, Johnstone F et al 1999a Uptake and acceptability of antenatal HIV testing. British Journal of Midwifery 7 (3): 151-156

Brahams D 1999 Court orders HIV 1 test for baby. Medico-Legal Journal 67 (3): 124-125

Brettle R P 2001 Injection drug use-related HIV infection. In: Adler M W (ed) The ABC of AIDS 5th edn. BMJ Books, London

British HIV Association 2001 British HIV Association (BHIVA) guidelines for the treatment of HIV infected adults with antiretroviral therapy. Available from www.bhiva.org/guidelines.htm Accessed 15 May 2002

Brocklehurst P, French R 1998 The association between maternal HIV infection and perinatal outcome: a systematic review of the literature and meta-analysis. British Journal of Obstetrics and Gynaecology 105: 836-848

Bruce M, Peacock J, Iversen A 2001 Hepatitis B and HIV antenatal screening 1: midwives' survey. British Journal of Midwifery 9 (8): 516-522

CDC 1992 1993 revised classification system for HIV infection and expanded surveillance case definition for AIDS among adolescents and adults. MMWR 41 (RR17): 1-19

CDC 1999 Appendix: Revised surveillance case definition for HIV infection. Available from www.cdc.gov/mmwr/preview/mmwrhtml/rr4813a2.htm Accessed 30 June 2002

CDSC Communicable Disease Surveillance Centre 2001 HIV and AIDS in the UK. An epidemiological review: 2000. Public Health Laboratory Service, London

CEM/CMO 1999 Antiretroviral drugs to reduce vertical transmission of HIV infection CEM/CMO/99/5 25 June 1999 Message from Professor A Breckenridge, Chairman of Committee on Safety of Medicines

Chippindale S, French L 2001 HIV counselling and the psychosocial management of patients with HIV or AIDS. In: Adler M W (ed) The ABC of AIDS 5th edn. BMJ Books, London

Chrystie I 1999 Screening of pregnant women: the case against [letter] Practising Midwife 2 (8): 38-39

Connor E M, Sperling R S, Gelber R et al 1994 Reduction of maternal-infant transmission of HIV type q with zidovudine treatment. New England Journal of Medicine 331: 1173-1180

Coutsoudis A, Pillay K, Kuhn L et al 2001 Method of feeding and transmission of HIV 1 from mothers to children by 15 months of age: prospective cohort study from Durban, South Africa. AIDS 15: 379-387

Darby S C, Ewart D W, Giangrande P L F et al 1996 Importance of age at infection with HIV 1 for survival and development of AIDS in UK haemophilia population. Lancet 347: 1573-1579

Davies S 2000 HIV universal voluntary testing in pregnancy – should midwives routinely recommend the test? MIDIRS Midwifery Digest 10 (3): 280-284

Department of Health 1992 Offering voluntary named HIV antibody testing to women receiving antenatal care. HMSO, London

Department of Health 1994 Guidance on offering voluntary confidential HIV testing during antenatal care. HMSO, London

Department of Health 1996 Guidelines for pre-test discussion on HIV testing. HMSO, London

Department of Health 1998 UK health departments guidance for clinical health care workers: protection against infection with blood-borne viruses. HMSO, London

Department of Health 1999 Reducing mother to baby transmission of HIV Health Service Circular 183

Department of Health 2000a Unlinked Anonymous Surveys Steering Group Prevalence of HIV and Hepatitis infections in the UK 1999. Department of Health, Public Health Laboratory Service, Institute of Child Health, Scottish Centre for Infection and Environmental Health

Department of Health 2000b Second report of the UK National Screening Committee. HMSO, London

Department of Health 2000c HIV post-exposure prophylaxis: Guidance from the UK Chief Medical Officer's Expert Advisory Group on AIDS (EAGA). HMSO, London

Department of Health 2001 Good Practice in Consent. Health Service Circular 23

Department of Health 2001a Unlinked Anonymous Surveys Steering Group. Prevalence of HIV and Hepatitis infections in the United Kingdom 2000. Department of Health, Public Health Laboratory Service, Institute of Child Health, Scottish Centre for Infection and Environmental Health

Department of Health 2001b HIV and infant feeding: guidance from the UK Chief Medical Officer's Expert Advisory Group on AIDS (EAGA). PL/CO (2001) 1 & PL/CNO (2001) 6

Department of Health 2001c New guidance on patient notification exercises when a health care worker is found to be infected with HIV [press release]. 28 November (2001/0574)

Department of Health 2001d Seeking consent – working with children. Available from www.doh.gov.uk/consent. Accessed 30 June 2002

Desmond N 1994 Knowledge about tests for HIV antibodies among pregnant women. British Medical Journal 309: 877

De Vincenzi I, for the European Study Group on Heterosexual Transmission of HIV 1994 A longitudinal study of human immunodeficiency virus transmission by heterosexual partners. New England Journal of Medicine 331: 341-346

Duffy T A, Wolfe C D A, Varden C et al 1998 Women's knowledge and attitudes, and the acceptability of voluntary antenatal HIV testing. British Journal of Obstetrics and Gynaecology 105: 849-854

Duffy T, Moore C 2000 Health visitors' knowledge and attitudes relating to HIV and AIDS. British Journal of Community Nursing 5 (9): 422-430

Dunn D T, Newell M L, Ades A E et al 1992 Risk of HIV type 1 transmission through breastfeeding. Lancet 340: 585-588

Dunn D T, Nicoll A, Holland F J et al 1995 How much paediatric HIV infection could be prevented by antenatal HIV testing? Journal of Medical Screening 2: 35-40

Duong T, Ades A E, Gibb D M et al 1999 Vertical transmission rates for HIV in the British isles: estimates based on surveillance data. British Medical Journal 319: 1227-1229

European Collaborative Study 1992 Risk factors for mother to child transmission of HIV 1. Lancet 339: 1007-1012

European Collaborative Study 1996 Vertical transmission of HIV 1: maternal immune status and obstetric factors. AIDS 10 (14): 1675-1681

European Collaborative Study 1998 Therapeutic and other interventions to reduce the risk of mother to child transmission of HIV 1 in Europe. British Journal of Obstetrics and Gynaecology 10: 704-709

European Mode of Delivery Collaboration 1999 Elective caesarean section versus vaginal delivery in prevention of vertical HIV 1 transmission: a randomised clinical trial. Lancet 353: 1035-1039

European Paediatric Hepatitis C Virus Network 2001 Effects of mode of delivery and infant feeding on the risk of mother to child transmission of hepatitis C virus. British Journal of Obstetrics and Gynaecology 108: 371-377

Food and Drug Administration 2001 Important drug warning – Zerit and Videx. Available from www.fda.gov/medwatch/safety/2001/zerit & videx_letter.htm. Accessed 30 May 2002

Forstein M 1984 The psychological impact of Acquired Immune deficiency Syndrome. Seminars in Oncology 11 (1): 72-82

French R, Brocklehurst P 1998 The effect of pregnancy on survival in women infected with HIV: a systematic review of the literature and meta-analysis. British Journal of Obstetrics and Gynaecology 105: 827-835

General Medical Council 2000 Confidentiality: protecting and providing information. Available from: www.gmc-org/standards/secret.htm. Accessed 6 September 2001

Gibb D M 1998a Guidelines for management of children with HIV infection. 3rd ed. AVERT, Horsham

Gibb D M, MacDonagh S E, Gupta R et al 1998 Factors affecting uptake of antenatal HIV testing in London: results of a multi-centre study. British Medical Journal 316: 259-261

Gill O N, Adler M W, Day N E 1989 Monitoring the prevalence of HIV. British Medical Journal 299: 1295-1298

Gilling-Smith C, Smith R J, Semprini A E 2001 HIV and infertility: time to treat. British Medical Journal 322: 566-567

Goedert J J, Duliege A M, Amos C I et al 1991 High risk of HIV 1 infection for first born twins. Lancet 338: 1471-1475

Goldberg D J, Johnstone F D 1993 Universal named testing of pregnant women for HIV. Lancet 306: 1144-1145

Grant A D, De Cock K 2001 HIV infection and AIDS in the developing world. In: Adler M W (ed) ABC of AIDS 5th edn. BMJ Books, London

Grellier R, Stears D, Clift S et al 1996 HIV/AIDS and midwifery: a study of knowledge, attitudes and practice among midwifery tutors, students and qualified midwives. Christchurch College, Canterbury

Grosskurth H, Mosha F, Todd J et al 1995 Impact of improved treatment of sexually transmitted diseases on HIV infection in rural Tanzania: randomised controlled trial. Lancet 346: 530-536

Guay L A, Musoke P, Fleming T et al 1999 Intrapartum and neonatal single dose nevirapine compared with zidovudine for prevention of mother to child transmission of HIV 1 in Kampala, Uganda: HIVNET 012 randomised trial. Lancet 354: 795-802

Harrison R, Corbett K 1999 Screening of pregnant women for HIV: the case against. The Practising Midwife 2 (7): 24-29

Hart R, Khalaf Y, Lawson R et al 2001 Screening for HIV, Hepatitis B and C in a population seeking assisted reproduction in an inner London hospital. British Journal of Obstetrics and Gynaecology 108: 654-656

HFEA 2001. Human Fertilisation and Embryology Authority Code of Practice 5th edn. HFEA, London

Intercollegiate Working Party 1998 Reducing mother to child transmission of

HIV infection in the United Kingdom. Royal College of Paediatrics and Child Health, London

International Perinatal HIV Group 1999 The mode of delivery and the risk of vertical transmission of HIV type 1. New England Journal of Medicine 340: 977-987

International Perinatal HIV Group 2001 Duration of ruptured membranes and vertical transmission of HIV 1: a meta-analysis from 15 prospective cohort studies. AIDS 15: 357-368

Ioannidis J P, Abrams E J, Amman A J et al 2001 Perinatal transmission of HIV type 1 by pregnant women with RNA virus loads < 1,000 copies/ml. Journal of Infectious Diseases 183 (4): 539-545

Johnstone F D 1996 HIV and pregnancy. British Journal of Obstetrics and Gynaecology 103: 1184-1190

Johnstone F, Brettle R, MacCallum L 1990 Women's knowledge of their antibody state: its effect on their decision whether to continue the pregnancy. British Medical Journal 300: 23-24

Jones S, Sadler T, Low N et al 1998 Does uptake of antenatal HIV testing depend on the individual midwife? Cross-sectional study. British Medical Journal 316: 272-273

Jungmann E, Edwards S, Booth T et al 2001 Is first trimester exposure to the combination of antiretroviral therapy and folate antagonists a risk factor for congenital abnormalities? Sexually Transmitted Infections 77 (6): 441-443

Justman J, Danoff A, Benning L et al 1999 Association of diabetes and protease inhibitor use in a large natural history cohort of HIV positive women. 6th conference on retroviruses and opportunistic infections, Chicago, IL. Jan/Feb Abstract 661

Kanki P J, Travers K U, Mboup S et al 1994 Slower heterosexual spread of HIV 2 than HIV 1. Lancet 343: 943-946

Kass N E, Taylor H A, Anderson J 2000 Treatment of HIV during pregnancy: the shift from an exclusive focus on fetal protection to a more balanced approach. American Journal of Obstetrics and Gynaecology 182: 856-859

Kovacs A, Wasserman S S, Burns D et al 2001 Determinants of HIV-1 shedding in the genital tract of women. Lancet 358: 1593-1601

Kuhn L, Abrams E L, Matheson P B 1997 Timing of maternal-infant HIV transmission: associations between intrapartum factors and early polymerase chain reaction results. AIDS 11: 429-435

Kulasegaram R, De Ruiter A 2001 An update on HIV infection. CME Urology 2 (3): 67-70

Kuppermann M, Gates E, Washington A E 1996 Racial-ethnic differences in prenatal diagnostic test use and outcomes: preferences, socio-economics or patient knowledge? Obstetrics and Gynaecology 87 (5): 675-682

Lallemant M, Jourdain G, Le Coeur S et al 2000 A trial of shortened zidovudine regimens to prevent mother to child transmission of HIV type 1. New England Journal of Medicine 343: 982-991

Lamey P J, Nolan A, Follett E A et al 1996 Anti HIV antibody in saliva: an assessment of the role of the components of saliva, testing methodologies and collection systems. Journal of Oral Pathology and Medicine 25 (3): 104-107

Landesman S H, Kalish L A, Burns D N et al 1996 Obstetrical factors and the transmission of HIV type 1 from mother to child. New England Journal of Medicine 334: 1617-1623

Larsson G, Spangberg L, Lindgren S et al 1990 Screening for HIV infection in pregnant women: a study of maternal opinion. AIDS Care 2 (3): 223-228

Laurent C 1995 A testing time. Health Professional Digest 9: 12-14

Lennette E H, Lennette D A, Lennette E T 1995 Diagnostic procedures for viral, rickettsial and chlamydial infections. American Public Health Association, Washington, DC

Lewis S H, Reynolds-Kohler C, Fox H E et al 1990 HIV 1 in trophoblastic and villous Hofbauer cells, and haematological precursors in eight week fetuses. Lancet 338 (8781): 1471-1475

Low N, Lambe C, Kennedy J et al 2001 HIV testing in antenatal care: a cross sectional study. British Journal of Midwifery 9 (6): 372-378

Lyall E G H, Blott M, de Ruiter A et al 2001 Guidelines for the management of HIV infection in pregnant women and the prevention of mother to child transmission. HIV Medicine 2: 314-334

Lyall E G H, Stainsby C, Taylor G P et al 1998 Review of uptake of interventions to reduce mother to child transmission of HIV by women aware of their HIV status. British Medical Journal 316: 268-270

Mandelbrot L, Mayaux M J, Bongain A 1996 Obstetric factors and mother to child transmission of HIV type 1: the French perinatal cohorts: SEROGEST and the French paediatric HIV infection study group. American Journal of Obstetrics and Gynaecology 175: 661-667

Manzini P, Saracco G, Cerchier A et al 1995 HIV infection as risk factor for mother to child hepatitis C virus transmission: persistence of anti hepatitis C virus in children is associated with the mother's anti hepatitis C virus immuno-blotting pattern. Hepatology 21: 328-332

Marcus S F, Avery S M, Abusheikha N et al 2000 The case for routine HIV screening before IVF treatment. A survey of UK IVF centre policies. Human Reproduction 15: 1657-1661

Markovitz D M 1993 Infection with the human immunodeficiency virus type 2. Annals of Internal Medicine 118: 211-218

Marteau T M, Slack J, Kidd J et al 1992 Presenting a routine screening test in antenatal care: oractice observed. Public Health 106: 131-141

Massiah H 1993 Antenatal testing may put pressure on women. British Medical Journal 36: 1753

Meadows J, Catalan J, Gazzard B 1993a HIV antibody testing in the antenatal clinic: the views of the consumers. Midwifery 9: 63-69

Meadows J, Catalan J, Gazzard B 1993b "I plan to have the HIV test" - predictors of testing intention in women attending a London antenatal clinic. AIDS Care 5 (2): 141-148

Meadows J, Jenkinson S, Catalan J 1994 Who chooses to have the HIV antibody test in the antenatal clinic. Midwifery 10: 44-48

Meadows J, Jenkinson S, Catalan J et al 1990 Voluntary testing in the antenatal clinic: differing uptake rates for individual counselling midwives. AIDS Care 2: 229-233

Mellors J, Rinaldo C R, Gupta P et al 1996 Prognosis in HIV 1 infection predicted by the quantity of virus in plasma. Science 272: 1167

Mercey D, Nicoll A 1998 We should routinely offer HIV screening in pregnancy. British Journal of Obstetrics & Gynaecology 105: 249-251

Miller R, Bor R, Dilley J W 1993 AIDS: a guide to clinical counselling. Science Press, Philadelphia and London

Mindel A, Tenant-Flowers M 2001 Natural history and management of early HIV infection. In: Adler M W (ed) ABC of AIDS 5th edn. BMJ Books, London

Minkoff H L, Landesman S H 1998 The case for routinely offering prenatal testing for human immuno-deficiency virus. American Journal of Obstetrics & Gynaecology 159: 793-796

Mofenson L 1994 Epidemiology and determinants of vertical HIV transmission. Seminars in Paediatric Infectious Diseases 5: 252-265

Mofenson L M 2001 Public health service task force recommendations for the use of antiretroviral drugs in pregnant women infected with HIV 1 for maternal health and for reducing perinatal HIV 1 transmission in the United States. Perinatal HIV Guidelines Working Group. CDC. May 4.

Mortimer P P, Loveday C 2001 The virus and the tests. In: Adler M W (ed) The ABC of AIDS 5th edn. BMJ Books, London

NAM 2000 Nutrition – Information series for positive people. NAM publication, London

Nduati R, John G, Mbori-Ngacha D et al 2000 Effect of breastfeeding and formula feeding on transmission of HIV 1. Journal of the American Medical Association 283: 1167-1174

Nduati R, Richardson B, John G et al 2000a Impact of breastfeeding on maternal mortality among HIV 1 infected women: results of a randomised clinical trial. 13th International Conference on AIDS abstract (WeOr C495) Durban 9-14 July 2000

Newman M D 1998 Primary care of women with HIV. Available from www.hivinsite.ucsf.edu/insite.jsp Accessed 1 May 2002

NHPIS (National HIV Prevention Information Service) 2001 HIV prevention and sexual health promotion with people with HIV. NHPIS Professional Briefing 4. Health Development Agency, London

Nicoll A, MacGarrigle C, Brady AR 1998 Epidemiology and detection of HIV 1 among pregnant women in the UK: results from national surveillance 1988-96. British Medical Journal 316: 253-258

Nicoll A, Newell M L, van Praag E et al 1995 Infant feeding policy and practice in the presence of HIV 1 infection. AIDS 9: 107-119

Pan London Local Authority Children and Families HIV Consultation Forum (Day E, Hamujuni-Smith B, Hart D) 2000 Child protection and HIV: recommendations for good practice. Pan London Local Authority Children and Families HIV Consultation Forum, London

Parekh B, Phillips S, Granade T et al 1999 Impact of HIV 1 subtype variation on viral RNA quantification. AIDS Res Human Retroviruses 15: 133-142

Parry J, Murphy G, Barlow K 2001 National Surveillance of HIV 1 subtypes for England & Wales: design, methods and initial findings. Journal of Acquired Immune Deficiency Syndrome.26: 381-388

PHLS (Public Health Laboratory Service) 1999 Occupational transmission of HIV: summary of published reports. Available from www.phls.co.uk/occupationaltransmission Accessed 18 May 2002

PHLS 1993 Case definition for AIDS – Europe and the United States part company. CDR Weekly 22 January

PHLS 2002 New data on AIDS and HIV published. CDR Weekly 31 January

Pillay K, Coutsoudis A, York D 2001 Cell free virus in breast milk of HIV 1 seropositive women. Journal of Acquired Immune Deficiency Syndrome 24: 330-336

Pizzo P A, Wilfert C M (eds) 1998 Pediatric AIDS: The challenge of HIV infection in infants, children and adolescents 3rd edn. Williams and Wilkins, Baltimore, MA

Positively Women 1994 Women like us: Positively Women's survey on the needs and experiences of HIV positive women. Positively Women Publications

Quinn T C, Wawer M J, Sewankambo N 2000 Viral load and heterosexual transmission of HIV type 1. Rakai Project Study Group. New England Journal of Medicine 342: 921-929

Reinisch J M, Hill C A, Sanders S A et al 1995 High-risk sexual behaviour at a midwestern university: a confirmatory survey. Family Planning Perspectives 27: 79-82

Richardson M P, Osrin D, Donaghy S et al 2000 Spinal malformations in the fetuses of HIV infected women receiving combination antiretroviral therapy and co-trimoxazole. European Journal of Obstetrics and Gynaecology and Reproductive Biology 93: 215-217

Romero J, Marincovich B, Castilla J et al 2002 Evaluating the risk of HIV transmission through unprotected orogenital sex. AIDS 16 (9): 1269-1297

Roth C, Feldman R, Lees S 2001 Antenatal HIV testing: a study of midwives' views and experiences. City University, London & South Bank University, London

Royal College of Midwives 1998 Position Paper 16a: HIV and AIDS. RCM, London

Royal College of Midwives 2002 HIV risk to asylum seekers' babies. RCM Midwives Journal 5 (4): 114

Royal College of Midwives and the Department of Health 2000 HIV and infant feeding: report of a seminar 30 June 2000. RCM, London

Royal College of Obstetricians and Gynaecologists 1997 HIV infection in maternity care and gynaecology: Working party report. RCOG, London

Royce R A, Sena A, Cates W J et al 1997 Sexual transmission of HIV. New England Journal of Medicine 336 (15): 1072-1078

Ruby C, Siney C 1997 Antenatal HIV antibody testing: a survey of maternity units in the UK. British Journal of Midwifery 5 (8): 493-495

Samson L, King S 1999 False positive results in antenatal HIV screening: the authors respond. Canadian Medical Association Journal 160: 1285

Scott K 2001 Lover found guilty of infecting girlfriend with HIV. The Guardian 24 February

Scoular A, Watt A D, Watson M et al 2000 Knowledge and attitudes of hospital staff to occupational exposure to bloodborne viruses. Communicable Disease and Public Health 3: 247-249

Semba R D, Miotti P G, Chiphangwi J D et al 1994 Maternal vitamin A deficiency and mother to child transmission of HIV 1. Lancet 343: 1593-1597

Semprini A E, Levi-Setti P, Bozzo M et al 1992 Insemination of HIV negative women with processed semen of HIV positive partners. Lancet 340: 1317-1319

Shaffer N, Chuachoowong R, Mock P A et al 1999 Short course zidovudine for perinatal HIV 1 transmission in Bangkok, Thailand: a randomised controlled trial. Lancet 353: 773-780

Sharland M 2001 Paediatric HIV infection. Medicine 29: 27-28

Sharland M, Castelli G, Ramos J T et al 2001a PENTA guidelines for the use of antiretroviral therapy in paediatric HIV infection. PENTA News, Summer

SHASTD (Society of Health Advisers in Sexually Transmitted Diseases) 2002 Partner notification guidelines. Available from www.shastd.org.uk. Accessed 7 May 2002

Sheon A R, Fox H E, Alexander G et al 1994 Misdiagnosed HIV infection in pregnant women: implications for clinical care. Public Health Reports 109: 694-699

Sherr L 1991 HIV and AIDS in mothers and babies: a guide to counselling. Blackwell Scientific, London

Sherr L, Barnes J, Elford J et al 1997 Women with HIV disease attending a London clinic. Genitourinary Medicine 73: 274-279

Sherr L, Bergenstrom A, Bell E et al 1998/9 Antenatal HIV screening and ethnic minority women. Health Trends 30 (4): 115-119

Sherr L, Hedge B 1990 The impact and use of written leaflets as a counselling alternative in mass antenatal HIV screening. AIDS Care 2 (3): 235-245

Sherr L, Jefferies S, Victor C et al 1996 Antenatal HIV testing: which way forward? Psychology, Health & Medicine 1 (1): 99-111

Simpson W M, Johnstone F D, Boyd F M et al 1998a Uptake and acceptability of antenatal HIV testing: randomised controlled trial of different methods of offering the test. British Medical Journal 316: 262-267

Simpson W M, Johnstone F M, Hart G J et al 1998b To test or not to test? What makes pregnant women decide to take an HIV test? Psychology, Health & Medicine 3 (3): 327-335

Siney C 1999 Pregnancy and drug misuse. Books for Midwives Press, Oxford

Smith D K, Shaw R W, Slack J et al 1995 Training obstetricians and midwives to present screening tests: evaluation of two brief interventions. Prenatal Diagnosis 15: 317-324

Smith N A, Shaw T, Berry N et al 2001 Antiretroviral therapy for HIV 2 infected patients. Journal of Infection 42 (2): 126-133

Smith N, Kennedy J, Bewley S et al 1998 HIV 2 in pregnancy: to treat or not to treat? International Journal of STD and AIDS 9: 246

Smith R, Dunlop J, Black S 1996 Antenatal screening for HIV in Scotland. Answer 23 AM-20 No 96/08

Stevens A, Victor C, Sherr L et al 1989 HIV testing in antenatal clinics. AIDS Care 1 (2): 165-171

Thirry L, Sprecher-Goldberger S, Jonckheer T 1985 Isolation of AIDS virus from cell-free breast milk of three healthy virus carriers. Lancet 2: 891

Towers C V, Deveikis A, Asrat T et al 1998 A "bloodless caesarean section" and perinatal transmission of the human immunodeficiency virus. American Journal of Obstetrics and Gynaecology 179: 708-714

Tudor-Williams G, Lyall E 1999 Mother to infant transmission of HIV. Current Opinion Infectious Diseases 12: 21-26

Tuomala R E, Shapiro D E, Mofenson L M et al 2002 Antiretroviral therapy during pregnancy and the risk of an adverse outcome. New England Journal of Medicine 346: 1863-1870

UK Association for Milk Banking Guidance for donors. Available at www.ukamb.org.donor.htm. Accessed 31 May 2002

UK Declaration of the Rights of People with HIV and AIDS. Available at www.nat.org.uk/docs/factsheet_6_human_rights.doc. Accessed 9 January 2003

UK Health Departments 1999 AIDS/HIV infected health care workers: guidance on the management of infected health care workers and patient notification. HMSO, London

UKCC (United Kingdom Central Council for Nursing, Midwifery and Health Visiting) 1992 Code of professional conduct. UKCC, London

UKCC (United Kingdom Central Council for Nursing, Midwifery and Health Visiting) 1996 Guidelines for professional practice. UKCC, London

UKCC (United Kingdom Central Council for Nursing, Midwifery and Health Visiting) 1998 Guidelines for records and record keeping. UKCC, London

UKCC (United Kingdom Central Council for Nursing, Midwifery and Health Visiting) 1998a Midwives rules and code of practice. UKCC, London

UNAIDS 2001 AIDS epidemic update. Available at www.unaids.org/epidemic_update/report

van de Perre P, Simonon A, Hitimana D 1993 Infective and anti-infective properties of breast milk from HIV infected women. Lancet 341: 914-918

van der Ende M E, Schutten M, Ly T D et al 1996 HIV 2 infection in 12 European residents: virus characteristics and disease progression. AIDS 10: 1649-1655

Weller I V D, Williams I G 2001 Treatment of infections and antiviral therapy. In: Adler M W (ed) ABC of AIDS 5th edn. BMJ Books, London

White J C 1997 HIV risk assessment and prevention in lesbians and women who have sex with women: practical information for clinicians. Health Care Women International 2: 127-138

Whittet S, Trail P, de Ruiter A et al 2000 General practitioners' attitudes and beliefs on antenatal testing for HIV: postal questionnaire survey. British Medical Journal 321: 934

WHO-UNAIDS HIV Vaccine Initiative. Available at www.who.int/HIV-vaccines. Accessed 30 May 2002

World Health Organization 2000 Preventing mother to child HIV transmission. Press Release WHO/70 from the WHO technical consultation. October 2000 www.who.int/inf-pr.2000/en/pr2000-70.html

Appendix I

AIDS defining conditions with laboratory evidence of HIV infection (CDC 1993)

Diseases diagnosed definitively

- Recurrent or multiple bacterial infections in child <13 years of age
- Coccidiomycosis – disseminated
- HIV encephalopathy
- Histoplasmosis – disseminated
- Isosporiasis with diarrhoea persisting >1 month
- Kaposi's sarcoma at any age
- Primary cerebral lymphoma at any age
- Non-Hodgkin's lymphoma: diffuse, undifferentiated B cell type, or unknown phenotype
- Any disseminated mycobacterial disease other than M tuberculosis
- Mycobacterial tuberculosis at any site
- Salmonella septicaemia – recurrent
- HIV wasting syndrome
- Recurrent pneumonia within one year
- Invasive cervical cancer

Diseases diagnosed presumptively

- Candidiasis – oesophagus
- Cytomegalovirus retinitis with visual loss
- Kaposi's sarcoma
- Mycobacteria disease (acid-fast bacilli; species not identified by culture) – disseminated
- Pneumocystis carinii pneumonia (PCP)
- Cerebral toxoplasmosis

Appendix 2

AIDS defining conditions without laboratory evidence of HIV (World Health Organization)

Disease defined definitively:

- Candidiais – oesophagus, trachea, bronchi or lungs
- Cryptococcosis – extrapulmonary
- Cryptosporidiosis with diarrhoea persisting >1 month
- Cytomegalovirus disease other than in liver, spleen, nodes
- Herpes simplex virus (HSV) infection: mucocutaneous ulceration lasting >1 month; pulmonary oesophageal involvement
- Kaposi's sarcoma in patient <60 years of age
- Primary cerebral lymphoma in patient <60 years of age
- Lymphoid interstitial pneumonia in child <13 years of age
- Mycobacterium avium – disseminated
- Mycobacterial kansasii – disseminated
- Pneumocystis carinii pneumonia
- Progressive multifocal leukoencephalopathy
- Cerebral toxoplasmosis

Appendix 3

HIV support groups and helplines

This is not an exhaustive list.

African AIDS Helpline
(English, French, Shona, Swahili and Luganda)
0800 0967 5000

African Community Involvement Association (ACIA)
Eagle Court, 224 London Road, Mitcham,
Surrey CR4 3HD
Administration: 020 8687 2400
Support groups, outreach and advocacy for African people.
Information on treatments, domiciliary support for home-bound
African people living with HIV/AIDS. Home and hospital visits.

Barnados Positive Options
William Morris Hall, 6 Somers Road, London E17 6RX
Phone: 020 8520 6625
Offers parents who are HIV positive the opportunity to plan for their
children's future, exploring options such as care by friends and relatives
as well as fostering.

Blackliners
Unit 46, Eurolink Centre, 49 Effra Road,
London SW2 1BZ
Administration: 020 7738 7468
Helpline: 020 7738 5274 (Mon-Fri 10am-8.30pm, Sat 1-6pm)

Body and Soul
9 Tavistock Place, London WC1H 9SN
Administration: 020 7383 7678
Runs support groups for women, children, heterosexual men, families
and young people living and affected by HIV and AIDS.

London East AIDS Network (LEAN)
35 Romford Road, London E15 4LY
Administration: 020 8519 9545
Advice and support service to people living with HIV and AIDS and those close to them. Includes support groups for women living with HIV and their children.

National AIDS Helpline
Helpline: 0800 567 123 (24 hours, free)
Support, information and referrals for everyone concerned about HIV.

National AIDS Manual (NAM) – Publications
16A Clapham Common Southside, London SW4 7AB
Phone: 020 7627 3200
NAM provides information both for professionals and organisations working in the fields and for individuals affected by HIV. Special rates are available for individuals, including free provision of NAM's monthly treatments newsletter and AIDS treatment update.

Positively Women
347-349 City Road, London EC1V 1 LR
Administration: 020 7713 0444
Direct Services: 020 7713 0222 (Mon-Fri 10am-4pm)
Positively Women is run for women by women with HIV and AIDS. Peer support services, individual counselling, home and hospital visits, helpline, support groups including a group for African women. Other services: information, welfare and housing advice, complementary therapies, children's worker.

The Terrence Higgins Trust Lighthouse
52-54 Grays Inn Road, London WC1X 8JU
THT Direct Helpline : 0845 1221200 (Mon-Fri 10am-10pm, Sat & Sun 12noon-6pm)
Administration: 020 7831 0330
Support and information provided on all aspects of living with HIV and AIDS including legal, welfare and housing advice. Services are available to people living with HIV and AIDS, their partners, family, friends and carers. The information centre holds a wide range of newsletters and journals on medical and complementary treatments plus free access to the Internet.

Uganda AIDS Action Fund (UAAF)
Unit K 1/2, Tower Bridge Business Complex, 100 Clement Road,
London SE16 4DG
Administration: 020 7394 8866
South London African Health Initiative (SLAHI): 020 7394 1005
*Support, advocacy and advice for Africans affected by HIV and AIDS
including advice on social and health services, accompanying people to
hospitals, social services and health departments.*

UK Coalition of People Living with HIV and AIDS
250 Kennington Lane,
London SE11 5RD
Phone: 020 7564 2180
Fax: 020 7564 2140
*Advocacy, activism, support and information for people living with
HIV and AIDS.*

Appendix 4

Useful resources

This is not an exhaustive list but, in conjunction with website addresses, support groups and helplines listed elsewhere, are resources the author has found useful in practice.

Video: HIV testing in pregnancy
Terrence Higgins Trust/Positively Women (see Appendix 3)

National AIDS manual
HIV and AIDS information source, regularly updated information, covering treatments and vaccines, transmission and prevention, referral and networking tools and the client's perspective.
NAM Publications (see Appendix 3)

HIV/AIDS treatment directory
Data on a wide range of issues including antiretroviral therapy, side effects, treatment failure, review of new drugs and data from major conferences.
NAM Publications (see Appendix 3)

Nambase
Information on all HIV related services in the UK in a database format. More than 1800 organisations listed including full contact details.
NAM Publications (see Appendix 3)

Appendix 5

Useful websites

This is not an exhaustive list and many of these sites will have links to other sources of information.

Aegis (AIDS Education Global Information Service)
www.aegis.com

AVERT (produce a range of information on HIV and AIDS)
www.avert.org

BHIVA (British HIV Association)
www.bhiva.org

Body and Soul
www.bodyandsoul.demon.co.uk

Centers for Disease Control and Prevention (HIV/AIDS prevention)
www.cdc.gov

Children with AIDS charity
www.cwac.org

Department of Health
www.open.gov.uk/doh/aids.htm

HIV/AIDS Treatment Information Service
www.aidsinfo.nih.gov

HIV Drug Interactions
www.hiv-druginteractions.org

HIV Insite Gateway to HIV and AIDS knowledge
http://hivinsite.ucsf.edu

HIV Nurses Association
www.NHIVNA.org.uk

Medscape's medpulse
www.medscape.com/hiv-aidshome

National AIDS Manual
www.aidsmap.com

National AIDS Trust
www.nat.org.uk

National HIV Prevention Information Service
www.hda-online.org.uk/nhpis

Paediatric HIV website
www.pedhivaids.org

PENTA (Paediatric European network for Treatment of AIDS)
www.ctu.mrc.ac.uk/penta

Positively Women
www.positivelywomen.org.uk

Public Health Laboratory service
www.phls.co.uk

SHASTD (Society of Health Advisors in Sexually Transmitted Diseases)
www.shastd.org.uk

Sigma Research (Community-based HIV research)
www.sigmaresearch.org.uk

Terrence Higgins Trust
www.tht.org.uk

UK Coalition of People Living with HIV and AIDS
www.ukcoalition.org

UNAIDS
www.unaids.org

World AIDS Day (December 1st)
www.worldAIDSday.org

World Health Organization
www.who.int

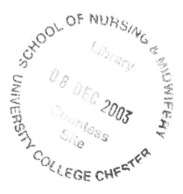

Index